Passing Your Advanced

# Passing Your Advanced Nursing OSCE

A guide to success in advanced clinical skills assessment

HELEN WARD
RN, BSc, DipNP, PGCert, PGCEA, MSc
*Principal Lecturer in Non-Medical Prescribing,*
*London South Bank University*

and

JULIAN BARRATT
RN, FHEA, BSc, PGCHE, MSc
*Senior Lecturer in Advanced Nursing,*
*London South Bank University*


*Foreword by*

JENNY ASTON
RN, RCNT, DipAsthma, BSc, PGDip
*Chair of the Royal College of Nursing*
*Nurse Practitioner Association*

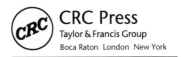

CRC Press
Taylor & Francis Group
Boca Raton  London  New York

CRC Press is an imprint of the
Taylor & Francis Group, an **informa** business

**Radcliffe Publishing Ltd**
St Mark's House
Shepherdess Walk
London
N1 7BQ

**www.radcliffehealth.com**

British Library Cataloguing in Publication Data
A catalogue record for this book is available from the British Library.

ISBN-13: 978 1 84619 234 0

Typeset by Pindar NZ, Auckland, New Zealand

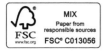

MIX
Paper from
responsible sources
FSC
www.fsc.org   FSC® C013056

# Contents

# List of tables and boxes

## Tables

## Boxes

# Foreword

No one who reads this book will be in any doubt that the expanding role of nurses is an important factor in the evolution of health services in the UK today. If we are to meet the growing demand for medical care from all segments of the population, nurses must take on additional responsibilities. Physical examination, history taking, prescribing and referrals were once the sole preserve of doctors, but each of these skills now forms part of advanced nursing practice. There are some in the medical community who doubt the wisdom of this development, so it is vital that those who practise at this level are properly trained and assessed to a consistent standard.

The objective structured clinical examination (OSCE) system effectively simulates genuine clinical situations and allows candidates to demonstrate whether they really are safe to practice at an advanced level. Having worked as an examiner on a number of different courses over many years, I am very aware that some students are much better prepared than others, so I welcome the publication of this book as a contribution towards raising the overall standard of advanced nursing practice and to achieving greater national consistency.

Both authors' backgrounds combine front-line clinical experience and many years of teaching and examining nurse practitioners and nurse prescribers at London South Bank University. The OSCE standard set by London South Bank University has influenced many other advanced practice programmes around the country. This very practical and well researched book will prove an invaluable resource for those preparing for OSCEs, whether as a student, examiner, or lecturer.

**Jenny Aston**
**Chair of the Royal College of Nursing Nurse Practitioner Association**
*October 2008*

# Preface

Registered nurses who wish to practise at a point beyond that of their initial registration, such as nurse practitioners, will normally undertake a specific undergraduate or postgraduate study course related to advanced clinical practice. A key element of these advanced nursing courses is the acquisition of advanced clinical practice skills by students and subsequent assessment of their advanced practice competence, most often utilising university-based practical examinations. This book aims to provide an easily accessible quick reference guide for advanced nursing students preparing to undertake their practical examinations for the assessment of advanced clinical practice competence, commonly known as an objective structured clinical examination (OSCE).

The OSCE is becoming an increasingly frequent method for assessing advanced nursing and prescribing clinical practice competence in the UK. However, the available study skills literature has not kept up with advanced nursing OSCE developments, and currently there is a lacuna in the provision of textbooks to assist both advanced nursing students and advanced nursing lecturers in preparing for their OSCEs. A number of OSCE study skills books exist that are aimed at medical students, but these all relate to the pre-registration level of medical education, and hence contain a mix of basic and advanced clinical practice skills. In contrast to medical students, advanced nursing students are all previously registered healthcare professionals, most often with many years of clinical experience behind them, they therefore do not need any preparation in basic clinical skills as they have already achieved these skills and have surpassed this level of attainment, by virtue of their post-registration status and subsequent clinical experience. However, as advanced nursing students need to develop their advanced clinical practice skills, this book seeks to directly address the preparation for OSCE-based assessment of nurse practitioners in advanced clinical practice skills.

We are both clinical academic nurse practitioners who regularly work in clinical practice in conjunction with teaching advanced nurse practitioner and non-medical prescribing students. We have extensive experience of preparing nurse practitioner and non-medical prescribing students for OSCEs, and in setting up and running OSCEs at BSc and MSc level through our work at the

Royal College of Nursing Institute and London South Bank University. Both these institutions were pivotal for the introduction of OSCEs in advanced nursing. This book utilises a case-study approach to present our experiences of using OSCEs for advanced nurse practitioner and non-medical prescribing assessment in a coherent, consistent, and easily understandable style. We hope this book will be incorporated and recommended as essential reading for many advanced nursing and non-medical prescribing programmes across the UK. It provides pertinent advice for advanced nursing students and academics alike; working from the context of an OSCE study skills guide specifically designed for advanced nursing students. Furthermore, it has been written by practising clinical academic nurse practitioners who are therefore conversant with the everyday reality of contemporary clinical practice.

**Julian Barratt**
**Helen Ward**
*October 2008*

# About the authors

**Helen Ward** has been working as a nurse practitioner since 1994 when she completed the Royal College of Nursing Nurse Practitioner Diploma. Helen works as a principal lecturer for both the non-medical prescribing and nurse practitioner programmes at London South Bank University. She also works clinically as a nurse practitioner in a nurse-led walk-in centre in central London.

**Julian Barratt** qualified as a registered nurse in 1991 and subsequently worked in emergency nursing. He has been working as nurse practitioner since 1997, in both secondary and primary health care settings. Julian works as a senior lecturer for the nurse practitioner programmes at London South Bank University. He also works clinically as a nurse practitioner in general practice in East Dulwich, London.

# Contributor

**Jaya Ahuja** MB BS MD
Senior Lecturer in Pharmacotherapeutics, London South Bank University. Dr Ahuja kindly contributed to sections of Chapter 9 (Non-medical prescribing OSCEs) and Chapter 10 (Marking the OSCE).

# Introduction

## How to use this book

This book focuses on the OSCE process as used for the assessment of advanced clinical practice competence for both BSc and MSc nurse practitioner students, and students undertaking non-medical prescribing programmes. It gives students step-by-step instructions on performing well in OSCE scenarios, and also gives guidance to academic staff on preparing for and marking OSCEs. Including advice for both students and lecturers in one guide may at first appear odd. However, we believe that the using OSCEs for assessing advanced practice competence should be an open and transparent process, with no behind the scenes preparation and assessment that is hidden from students. Indeed, it is hoped that some students, depending on their learning style, may find the inclusion of this type of insider background information useful for their OSCE revision.

This book must be viewed solely as an advanced nursing and non-medical prescribing OSCE preparation and revision text, and not as a guide for clinical practice. Each university will recommend a core clinical textbook to guide student learning and their own teaching of history taking and physical examination skills. This preparation and revision book should be read in conjunction with any recommended core clinical textbooks in each respective university. This is an important consideration, as the recommended core clinical textbook normally informs the OSCE marking criteria for each individual university and accordingly students should be aware of this correlation. The core clinical textbook which has influenced the content of this book is *Bates' Guide to Physical Examination and History Taking.*[1]

This book comprises 10 chapters related to the OSCE process for advanced clinical practice assessment in nursing and non-medical prescribing. It is not intended to be read straight through in its entirety. Instead, each chapter can be read as an individual section, depending on the type of preparation or revision information required. Each chapter starts with a brief commentary on the type of OSCE station presented, which is followed by summary sequences for the skills required and related examples of OSCE station marking criteria. The actual style of presentation of the OSCE marking criteria may vary from university to university, though the content of the stations will generally be similar with small differences being guided by each university's recommended core clinical textbook.

## Reference

1 Bickley L, Szilagyi P. *Bates' Guide to Physical Examination and History Taking*. 9th ed. London: Lippincott; 2007.

# 1

# Introduction to the OSCE process

## The advanced nursing OSCE examination

The advanced nursing objective structured clinical examination (OSCE) is a structured assessment of specific clearly defined clinical skills. In this exam students complete a sequence of practical examinations designed to assess separate components of a consultation requiring the use of advanced clinical practice skills, such as history taking and physical examination.

The OSCE was first developed as a method of assessment to objectively measure the clinical competence of medical students in the late 1970s.[1] Their development was in response to a recognition that the more traditional methods of assessment, such as written examinations and essays, whilst reflecting academic attainment, did not always test clinical competence. Consequently it was recognised that a formal assessment of clinical skills that moved beyond informally testing clinical skills at the bedside was required. While the OSCE is now an established method of clinical assessment for medical education, it has taken rather longer to be adopted for assessing clinical skills in nursing. However, it has recently gained in popularity and is now widely used to assess advanced clinical competence in students such as registered nurses preparing to become either nurse practitioners or nurse independent prescribers. The OSCE can be a valuable educational tool when used alongside other traditional methods of assessment, such as essays or exams, bringing together both clinical and academic strands of the educational development of advanced nursing students.

The advanced nursing OSCE is a practical assessment of advanced clinical skills. In this students complete a set of individual OSCE stations (individual

OSCEs are normally called 'stations') that are designed to test a range of clinical skills used in patient consultations, with an examiner using a previously determined, objective scoring scheme. A group of collated OSCE stations to be used in actual student examinations is called an OSCE 'session'. The students are not normally aware of the actual planned station topic content of an OSCE session, as OSCEs, in line with traditional written examinations, are normally attempted as unseen examinations, to mirror the uncertainty of everyday clinical practice.

## History of OSCE usage in advanced nursing

Building on the success of OSCEs in undergraduate medical education, the Royal College of Nursing Institute nurse practitioner programme first pioneered the use of the OSCE in advanced nursing, beginning in the early 1990s. This innovative, but often controversial, programme pushed the boundaries of nursing from the traditional 'handmaiden', task-orientated approach into a more modern one; integrating critical questioning and clinical problem solving in a clearly defined curriculum of advanced clinical skills. While developing this programme, it became clear that an objective practical assessment strategy was needed to assess the clinical competence of the student nurse practitioners who were developing the advanced clinical skills of history taking, physical examination and clinical reasoning; skills that were previously solely within the remit of the medical profession.

The OSCE was adapted from the original medical student model in order to assess the clinical competence of the nurse practitioner students at the Royal College of Nursing Institute. This original nurse practitioner OSCE was developed as a session of 10 stations, each of 10 minutes duration, which included two written stations and eight simulated patient scenarios. These stations were initially developed to reflect the advanced clinical skills taught in the classroom and then developed in clinical practice. This 10-station model proved successful and a variant of it is still used today by the former Royal College of Nursing Institute nurse practitioner team, which was transferred to the RCN Development Centre at South Bank University in 2000, and laterally to London South Bank University in 2003.

Now other universities across the UK, in common with the Royal College of Nursing Institute and London South Bank University, also train registered nurses wanting to practise nursing at an advanced level using structured programmes of post-registration advanced nursing education. These programmes usually comprise units pertaining to advanced clinical practice, such as physiology, clinical examination, consultation communication skills, clinical diagnosis, pharmacology, prescribing and patient management. All these clinically focused units are assessed from a traditional academic perspective.

However, it is not sufficient to assess students' attainment in these clinical units solely on an academic basis, as these units are specifically designed to help students develop practically orientated advanced nursing skills, which are required for competent clinical practice as a nurse practitioner. Consequently, other universities have also started to use OSCE-based practical assessments of students' acquisition of advanced clinical practice skills, and their subsequent development of advanced practice competence. Different OSCE models have been adapted over the years to meet the challenges faced by advanced nurse educators for the most appropriate way to assess clinical competence in advanced nursing students. While the format of advanced nursing OSCEs varies across universities, they all share the principle of seeking to objectively assess a student's proficiency in common advanced clinical practice skills such as history taking and physical examinations.

The OSCE process is now also widely used in pre-registration nursing to assess fundamental clinical skills, such as recording and interpreting vital signs. In contrast, advanced nursing OSCEs assess the clinical performance of post-registration nurses, as opposed to novice pre-registration nurses, and therefore do not include assessments of basic clinical skills such as recording vital signs, because pre-validated attainment of these skills is implicit in a nurse practitioner student's professional registration as a qualified nurse. Instead, assessment of the combined experiential, practical and theoretical clinical skills at the competent or proficient level of advanced nursing practice is required.[2] As such, advanced nursing OSCEs assess a level of clinical complexity beyond that required of an initial registrant in nursing, and therefore carefully planned, consistent, and sustained OSCE preparation is required throughout a nurse practitioner degree programme on the parts of both students and academic staff. Student and lecturer OSCE preparation is discussed in more detail in chapters 2 and 3 respectively.

## Do OSCEs assess clinical safety or role competence?

Whether OSCEs assess clinical safety or role competence is an area of debate. If we strictly adhere to inflexible parameters for safe practice, a student could potentially, in the name of safety, refer every patient they see to either a medical practitioner or a specialist nurse for a second opinion. While this may be a safe practice, it does not conform to the everyday level of independent practice realistically required from an advanced nurse practitioner to assess, plan, deliver and evaluate patient care. Therefore, there is a baseline at which we expect an advanced nurse to operate. Students need to demonstrate their ability to work bounded by the limits of their advanced role competence within an overall safe approach. Accordingly, students need to be able to identify potentially serious clinical signs and symptoms in their OSCE stations, and conversely OSCE stations need to be designed to give students an opportunity to identify serious clinical signs and symptoms. In response to our question advanced nursing OSCEs should seek to assess both clinical safety and role competence.

## Validity of the OSCE process

The term 'validity' refers to the extent to which a measurement actually measures what it is intended to (i.e., does the OSCE do what it says its does?). The validity of the OSCE as an examination process is necessary, as universities are obliged to produce advanced nursing graduates capable of working in the role for which they are being assessed, whether this is an advanced nurse practitioner, or a nurse independent prescriber.

OSCEs comprise two types of validity: content validity and face validity. The *content validity*, in relation to the OSCE, is judged by a panel of experts about the range which the content of the examination appears to coherently examine, and includes the characteristics and domains that it is designed to appraise and assess.[3] Content validity is addressed by regularly reviewing the process through which OSCE stations are developed and their content is updated. The content of the OSCE must reflect the curricular content taught on the programme for which the OSCE forms the practical clinical assessment. An OSCE specification table, which explicitly indicates where the core clinical practice skills are assessed in each OSCE station helps to ensure validity, via cross-referenced demonstration of programme learning outcomes.

*Face validity* addresses the question of whether the marking criteria actually measure what they are intended to measure. For example, if the marking criteria requirements of a station are too difficult for the students to answer successfully, or cannot be completed in the allocated time for the station, then its inclusion needs to be reviewed.

## Reliability of the OSCE process

The test score obtained is reliable if it gives a reasonable indication of a student's performance in that particular test (i.e., are the OSCE scores consistently related to students' performances?). The criterion of reliability implies that the OSCE is a stable, predictable and dependable method of assessment. Several factors may influence the reliability of the OSCE: the demeanour of students and examiners and their subsequent interactions; subjective interpretations on the part of the examiners; and environmental factors, such as the examination room, noise levels, light and temperature.

The issue of examiner subjectivity can be addressed through the use of an independent OSCE examiner who observes the conduct of the examiner at each station to monitor the fairness and consistency of the examiners' decisions. One key factor influencing the reliability of the OSCE is its length. As the number of items being assessed is increased, the chance factors influencing the score are reduced, thus giving a better estimate of the true score the student is likely to achieve, which in turn, increases the reliability of the OSCE.[4]

## Range of advanced nursing skills typically assessed in an OSCE session

Most advanced nurse practitioner OSCEs are specially designed to test the range of competencies specific to advanced clinical practice, as described in the domains and competencies for advanced nurse practitioner practice developed by the Royal College of Nursing from those originally published in the USA by the National Organisation of Nurse Practitioner Faculties.[5] Accordingly, the ranges of advanced clinical practice skills typically assessed by OSCEs are:

- interpersonal and communication skills
- history-taking skills
- physical examination of specific body systems
- mental health assessment
- clinical decision making, including the formation of differential diagnosis
- clinical problem-solving skills
- interpretation of clinical findings and investigations
- management of a clinical situation, including treatment and referral
- patient education
- health promotion
- acting safely and appropriately in an urgent clinical situation.

At London South Bank University we test our final-year undergraduate nurse practitioner student attainment in these ranges of advanced clinical practice skills by using a 10-station OSCE session which comprises three physical examination stations; three history-taking stations; three stations that cover communication skills, conveying information, and treatment and management; and, finally, one question and answer station, usually looking at the students' responses to an urgent clinical situation. These station areas are chosen to test the scope of advanced clinical knowledge and skills that may be applied across the age range in primary healthcare settings. For our postgraduate nurse practitioner students, we use a two-station long case OSCE-style session, which examines in the more detail the students' depth of advanced clinical knowledge, as opposed to their breadth of knowledge, such as is tested in the 10-station OSCE session. However, these OSCE session examples are drawn solely from London South Bank University, and there is a wide variance in the amount and type of OSCE stations used in OSCE sessions in other universities across the UK. One OSCE session format is not necessarily more correct than another, as all advanced nursing OSCEs should have the ultimate goal of testing students' attainment of the domains and competencies for advanced nurse practitioner practice.

## References

1 Harden R, Gleeson F. Assessment of clinical competence using an objective structured clinical examination (OSCE). *Med Educ.* 1979; 13: 41–54.
2 Waldner M, Olson J. Taking the patient to the classroom: applying theoretical frameworks to simulation in nursing education. *Int J Nurs Educ Scholarsh.* 2007; 4(1): 1–14.
3 Bowling A. *Research Methods in Health: investigating health and health services.* Buckingham: Open University Press; 2002.
4 Burns R. *Introduction to Research Methods.* London: Sage; 2000.
5 Royal College of Nursing. *Advanced Nurse Practitioners: an RCN guide to the advanced nurse practitioner role, competencies and programme accreditation.* London: Royal College of Nursing; 2008.

## Further reading

Rushforth H. Objective structured clinical examination (OSCE): review of literature and implications for nursing education. *Nurse Educ Today.* 2007; 27: 481–90.
Ward H, Barratt J. Assessment of nurse practitioner advanced clinical practice skills: using the objective structured clinical examination (OSCE). *Primary Health Care.* 2005; 15(10): 37–41.

# 2

# OSCE study skills for students

This chapter discusses relevant study skills that should guide you as a student through the OSCE process so you can feel confident when you come to take your OSCE. Most universities that use an OSCE as part of the assessment process will prepare a study guide to support you with the OSCE. You must read your own university's guide and become familiar with its contents, as it will explain the practical parts of the OSCE process as applied in your university.

## The OSCE as an examination

For success in OSCEs you need to recognise that the OSCE is an actual examination. This means that you must actually learn and revise the relevant information to employ in your OSCE, exactly as you do in a traditional written examination. It is not enough to merely read your course's recommended clinical textbook and related lecture notes to pass an OSCE. Students who only do this level of preparation are often referred. You need to actively take in this information by learning and committing to your mind summary sequences for history taking and physical examination. It is only when you have learned these summary sequences that you will be able to demonstrate confidence during an actual OSCE.

As the OSCE is a practical skill you must also be sure to practise the requisite skills in your practice setting both with and without supervision from your facilitator or mentor. In addition to learning in your clinical setting it can also help to practise OSCE skills informally in small groups with your student peers. This type of small group learning can be undertaken in a more relaxed style and allows you to discuss and develop your skills with others who are preparing for the same assessment.

## The OSCE as role-play

A further step for success in OSCEs is that you need to realise that they require a certain amount of role-play on the parts of examiners, patients and students. You should therefore, as far as possible, present yourself professionally as you would do in your normal day-to-day clinical practice. By this we are not referring to your appearance, but instead to your demonstration of calm, confident and courteous professional interactions. So you should interact with the examiner and patient as much as possible as you would do when working in practice, which also emphasises the importance of practising OSCE skills in your clinical setting. It is often very easy for examiners to spot students who appear uncertain in their interactions, which can affect their overall assessment of an OSCE performance. Remember that part of the skills required of the advanced practitioner is being able to demonstrate the impression of confident practice, even when faced with clinical uncertainty.

## Practicalities of the OSCE process

Individual OSCEs are most often presented as time-limited stations. This time can range from 5 minutes to one hour or more. Find out the time limits that will be used for your university's OSCEs. You will normally be given a time indicator (such as an alarm or a verbal warning) before the end of an OSCE station. This helps you to know whether you need to speed up or if you are on track for successfully completing a station.

Most OSCE stations will normally comprise three people: you, the examiner and the patient. During a station you should address, as required, both the examiner and the patient. Examiner roles are normally undertaken by course lecturers, qualified nurse practitioners or medical doctors; all of whom should be familiar with the OSCE process of your university. Patient roles can also be undertaken by course lecturers or qualified clinicians, but actors are sometimes also used to play the role of patients. It is also possible that actual patients may be used in advanced OSCEs, though this happens less often in comparison to the usage of real patients by the medical royal colleges for their professional membership exams.

As regards performing in an OSCE station, remember that in physical examination stations you will actually be required to examine the person playing the role of the patient. This means that this person will need to selectively undress, as required for an examination. However the patients will not do this by themselves; they will wait for you to ask them to get undressed. You will also need to make appropriate use of the diagnostic equipment placed at your station, so you should make yourself familiar, before an OSCE, with equipment such as stethoscopes and otoscopes. It is possible that the person playing the role of patient may have underlying medical pathologies which may or may not be related to their OSCE station. If, on examination, you note a possible pathological abnormality you should report this to the examiner for your station.

## Formative OSCEs

You may find that that you are given OSCE preparation throughout the advanced nursing programme you are studying on; for example, you may have a mock OSCE as a formative assessment. Here the feedback from your OSCE should be constructive and should be given to you as soon as possible after you have undertaken the mock OSCE, while it is still fresh in your mind, so as to inform your future clinical skills development. Listen to what the examiner has to tell you. The feedback should be around your communication skills as well as your knowledge base. The 'patient' may want to give you feedback about how they felt as the patient, for example, did you make them feel comfortable? Were you listening to what they were saying or were you just asking rote learned questions? Did you give them time to ask you questions? The formative OSCE gives you the opportunity to understand the OSCE process under exam conditions and to grasp the structure of the OSCE paper, so that when you come to do the real OSCE exam you will know exactly what to do from a practical perspective.

## Some tips for OSCE preparation

### Preparatory tips

- Consider what clinical scenarios may come up. Listen carefully to your lecturers: they may (inadvertently) give you a hint!
- Consider the necessary knowledge and skills that you need to have to complete the OSCE. These requirements should be presented in the university documents related to the OSCE process.

### History taking tips

- Memorise the key points involved in taking an effective (structured and systematic) history.
- Consider using an *aide mémoire* such as a mnemonic device when practising taking a history to ensure that you do not omit any key points.
- Practise taking a history in the time allowed for you. For example, if you have 10-minute history-taking station, practise taking the history in

10 minutes. Use a clock or a timer so that you have a good sense of how long or short 10 minutes can be, and what you can realistically achieve in a limited time period.

- Practise on family and friends, as well as patients, until you feel confident in taking a history in a systematic structured manner, while at the same time demonstrating good communication skills with your patient. Your patients should not feel that they are being barracked with questions.

### Physical examination tips

- Consider which physical examinations you may be expected to perform in the OSCE.
- Memorise the normal physical examination sequence expected for each physical examination system.
- Practise the physical examination of each system in the time allowed, for example, 10 minutes. Use a clock or a timer as a guide for your timing.
- Some physical examinations may only take you a few minutes to perform, so ensure these are done thoroughly and systematically.
- Practise explaining what you are doing, what you are feeling/listening for and thinking as you perform the physical examination.
- You should be prepared to explain what abnormal findings could be elicited from your physical examination, and what these might mean in terms of differential diagnoses.

### OSCE communication skills tips

- Revise the key principles of effective communication, health education, explaining a result, decision making and prioritising, effectively managing an urgent clinical scenario, and working with feelings and emotions. If there are areas of clinical communication in which you do not feel confident, or are not common situations within your area of clinical practice, you should practise these communication skills with colleagues, friends, or family until you feel more confident.

### Tips for practising OSCE stations

- Remember that you can practise stations by role-playing and discussing possible scenarios with your peers, facilitator or colleagues at work.
- Do not decide not to practise for a station because you are not familiar with its content; it could come up in an OSCE.
- It is not acceptable to say in an OSCE 'this is not my area of practice; I will refer this patient on'. If the subject area has been taught during your course, then it could be included as an OSCE station.

- Sometimes, there is a tendency to rush things, especially when you are anxious or nervous. Ten minutes can seem a long time when you are practising, but it will go very quickly when you are in the actual exam.

## On the day of the OSCE: guidance and tips

The OSCE is your opportunity to demonstrate the clinical skills and knowledge that you have learnt while undertaking the programme you are on. You will be nervous and the examiners will be aware of this and will do everything possible to alleviate your nerves. Be well prepared and know exactly where you have to be and at what time. There is nothing worse than getting even more flustered because you are late. Arrive on time and let the OSCE co-ordinator know that you are here.

The OSCE co-ordinator may wish to have an OSCE briefing with you and your student colleagues before you start your OSCE. Listen carefully to what they say. The instructions that you are given will be important and may include:

- housekeeping arrangements: fire exits, fire alarms, toilets, breaks in the OSCE and rules on entering and leaving a station
- your initial start station
- the order in which the OSCE is run
- the time of each individual station
- the type of stations. For example, in a 10-station OSCE there may be three history-taking stations, three physical examination stations and four other types of station, such as communication, conveying information, and treatment and management
- any rest intervals that you may be required to take from stations
- the equipment you might need to undertake the OSCE and the equipment available at individual stations
- the use of evidence-based guidelines or drug formularies during an OSCE
- making notes while you are in the OSCE
- what to do if you finish before the allotted time
- why it is important not to discuss station content between stations with your colleagues
- what to do if you get upset during the OSCE
- how the station timing is indicated to you. For example, if the stations are 10 minutes long, the OSCE co-ordinator may let you know when eight minutes have passed and that you have two minutes left to complete the station
- what to do if you leave the station before the time for the OSCE station is

up. If at all possible you should try and remain at a station until the end of the allotted time, as you may suddenly remember any omissions in your performance that you may wish to rectify with the examiner
- whether you have an opportunity to ask any questions of the OSCE co-ordinator before you start the OSCE.

---

### Three essential summary tips for OSCE revision

1 Ensure you are aware of the assessment regulations and requirements for your university's OSCEs, including the range and breadth of the OSCEs you will need to complete.
2 Learn and revise (i.e., commit to memory) potential OSCE station sequences.
3 Practise OSCE station sequences in your clinical setting, with student peer group colleagues and, informally, with family or friends.

---

## Further reading

Franklin P. How to ensure you pass an OSCE. *Nurs Times.* 2005; 101(43): 76–7.

# 3

# OSCE preparation for academic staff

## How to develop an OSCE station

OSCE station development varies from university to university, and so far there is no national standard OSCE format for advanced nursing practice education. A fundamental concern in OSCE development is to ensure that the planned station content reflects the teaching content of its related academic unit, and that the marking criteria for a station should correspond with the learning outcomes of the associated programme or unit.

The generation of ideas for an OSCE station may come from the academic team. For example, a member of the academic team may want to develop a specific station related to musculoskeletal examination. To develop this station the lecturer must consult appropriate up-to-date evidence-based literature, and if they are not a subject specialist or clinically experienced in the topic of the proposed OSCE station, consultation with a clinical expert is ideally required. Once the station has been drafted it then needs to be developed and piloted before it can be used live in an OSCE. Student or examiner OSCE workshops provide ideal opportunities for OSCE station piloting, as the end users of potential stations can then provide a critical review of the proposed station content and format.

Once the OSCE station has been developed and piloted it should be scrutinised by a panel of experts, which should include an external examiner and at least one expert from the clinical area in which the OSCE scenario is based. The finally selected marking criteria should be cross-referenced against the university's core clinical textbook and any national policy guidelines. The commissioned OSCE stations should then be kept up to date and regularly reviewed by the academic team running the OSCE.

Not only do the marking criteria have to be evidence-based, clear and accurate, but so do the student instructions, patient instructions and examiner instructions. If the instructions are not clear, the student, patient or examiner may misinterpret them and either, in the case of students, not answer the question correctly, or, in the case of an examiner or patient, run the station incorrectly. If the marking criteria or station instructions are not clear and explicit, then the examiner may make subjective decisions about the students' competence. Such decisions may vary from student to student and so alter the reliability of the station. The marking criteria must be clear enough to enable the examiner to indicate whether the student has fulfilled the criteria either correctly, incorrectly or not at all. This marking scheme can take several different forms. One of the most straightforward OSCE station scoring systems is to rate each individual marking criterion using one of the following categories:

- done correctly
- not done correctly
- not done at all/omitted.

OSCE scoring and marking is considered in more detail in chapter 10.

## How to prepare students for the OSCE

As previously mentioned, successful performance at an OSCE requires sustained preparation on the part of the student throughout their course of study. Advanced nursing clinical academic staff play a key role in supporting students for this sustained preparation. Provision of OSCE information is an essential activity which should start right at the beginning of a course and continue until the OSCEs have been completed. Students should receive a mix of verbal, documentary and online information to support their OSCE educational development. Verbal and documentary information can be provided in time-tabled classroom sessions dedicated to OSCE preparation so that students are made aware of OSCE requirements from the beginning of their course.

Most advanced nursing courses start with an introductory clinical examination unit and it is at this initial interval that small-scale OSCE examinations should be introduced so that students can gain experience of the OSCE process as soon as possible. At this initial stage the OSCEs can either be formative or summative, dependent on individual course requirements. As students progress towards the completion of a course the OSCEs should move definitively towards a purely summative assessment with a wider range of possible OSCE stations.

A practically focused method of student support is to run regular OSCE preparation workshops. In these workshops students can be informed of the exact requirements for their particular OSCEs, practical arrangements can be made (such as allocating students to station times), and students can have the opportunity to ask questions about the OSCE in peer groups. Lecturers should ensure during these workshops that no student is unclear about the practicalities and format of the impending OSCEs, so they are not disadvantaged in their prospective performance.

Once these practical considerations have been attended to, another activity that can be undertaken in an OSCE preparation workshop is supervised student practice of mock OSCE stations under simulated exam conditions. Students can be placed in small groups of three individuals, rotating in the respective roles of student, patient and examiner, and using actual OSCE exam papers and scenarios as a guide. At the end of the station rotation the supervising clinical academic staff can briefly review the students' progress and answer any further questions that may have arisen from their performance of the station. In our experience students invariably find these practically focused workshop sessions greatly beneficial and reassuring for their OSCE preparation and subsequent examination performance.

## Using video recorded simulated OSCEs for student preparation

A common student request at OSCE preparation workshops is for the lecturing team themselves to perform a mock OSCE station in front of the class group so that the students can see how they can practically complete and successfully pass an OSCE. While such requests are understandable and appropriate, it is resource intensive to stage a simulated OSCE as it requires at least two members of staff, and it can also be difficult to give a coherent 'live' OSCE performance in front of a typical workshop group size of up to 30 advanced nursing students.

In light of these requests for live OSCE performances, and their staff and time demands, we have considered alternative methods of meeting the students' OSCE learning needs. In both nurse practitioner and general practitioner consultation, video recorded simulated clinical consultations have been used for educational development purposes and have often been favourably evaluated. Video recordings have been applied in medical education and research since the mid-1980s; particularly for evaluating and learning consultation communication skills.[1,2] Video recordings have recently gained increased popularity in other academic disciplines, such as nursing and education, due to the verified usefulness of medical education videos for professional development, and also the increasing ease of use of video camcorders and their recent transition to digital media.[3]

Given this prior educational success, the use of simulated video recordings as an OSCE educational preparation method was adopted and developed by our clinical academic team. Video recording as a support method for OSCE educational development is appealing for the following reasons: digital camcorder technology is easy to use; video recording allows staff resources and time to be used flexibly; OSCE performance mistakes can be rectified; the same video recordings can be used with multiple cohorts of students and, because recordings are digital, they can be made available via video streaming on Internet-based platforms such as a university's virtual learning environment or publicly available video sharing sites such as You Tube, which means students are able to access the recordings at any convenient time.

We initially produced a preliminary video recording of one history-taking OSCE station, which was piloted with final-year nurse practitioner students. Reflecting on this recording we noted it was largely unscripted; there was no introduction and it did not 'look right', as it had not been recorded in a skills lab (where the students' OSCEs normally take place). However, when this recording was shown to the final-year students, it was well evaluated, so this spurred us on to improve our later attempts at recording a simulated OSCE. To aid this improvement we consulted the work of Corbally,[4] who has presented some tips on producing nursing education clinical skills videos. Corbally's[5] main recommendations are to ensure that the planned script fits the available time (we achieved this through using the actual scenario criteria for some of our 10-minute OSCE stations); filming the video in a 'nursing skills centre' (we recorded the subsequent videos in a university clinical skills lab) and ensuring access to appropriate video recording equipment (which was available to us as a JVC Everio GZ-MG77EK Hard Disk Camcorder, offering digital video recording and uploading). We have now recorded a range of simulated OSCEs covering areas such as cough history taking, ear, nose and throat examination, abdominal examination and history taking, knee examination, back pain history taking, and paediatric fever assessment.

Our students have reported, via focus group evaluations, that the simulated OSCE video recordings fulfil their main learning style preference for visual learning; provide them with clarification of OSCE details that they are unclear about; reinforce their class-based OSCE learning and give them reassurance. In particular they find that the online availability of the video recordings is very useful, as they can revisit the learning materials in their own time and use them at their own speed.

These videos are an ongoing project and we urge other universities to use similar video recorded simulated OSCEs to support the learning needs of advanced nursing students. Our current selection of simulated OSCE video recordings can be viewed at http://www.youtube.com/LSBUOSCE.[6]

## How to set up and run a successful OSCE session

The OSCE is an expensive, time-consuming, labour-intensive examination. The key to running a successful OSCE session is for the academic, technical and administrative staff responsible to be well briefed, organised, and prepared for most eventualities. The following section focuses on the OSCE co-ordinator's role, as this is the key role for setting up and running a successful OSCE session.

### Preparation for an OSCE session

An OSCE session will normally run smoothly if an OSCE co-ordinator is allocated to take full responsibility for the organisation of the OSCE. This role is demanding and requires the co-ordinator to be well prepared for the OSCE event. Preparation for an OSCE should ideally start approximately three months before the OSCE is due to take place. The co-ordinator will need to decide how many stations and what type of stations the OSCE requires. This will depend on the programme being assessed and the level of the OSCE. Liaison with other members of the academic team will be required to decide upon the final selection of stations.

Once the date, time, format and content of the OSCE has been agreed, potential OSCE examiners and patients will need to be contacted and their availability established. This can be done by letter or e-mail. Make sure the deadline date for replies is included, and allow enough flexibility to contact alternative participants in the event of any negative replies.

The OSCE co-ordinator will then need to ensure that all the OSCE stations have the required examiner and 'patient', and that patient scenarios are allocated appropriately. For example, if the OSCE scenario requires a young female 'patient' presenting with acute abdominal pain, the simulated patient must be played by a young woman. Similarly, if the OSCE scenario requires the patient to be of a specific ethnic origin, try to ensure the role of the patient is played by a person with a corresponding ethnic background.

Once the co-ordinator has matched the examiners and patients to the stations it is advisable to reconfirm the availability and suitability of the examiners and patients before the planned OSCE session. Here you are establishing an informal contract with the examiners and role-playing patients.

Try to ensure that participants confirm their availability, as being let down by either examiners or patients at the last minute can be very frustrating. One way of minimising last-minute cancellations is to issue a confirmatory letter saying that OSCE session non-attendance should occur only for serious circumstances such as bereavement, illness or injury, or transport disruptions.

Two to three weeks before the OSCE is due to take place, the co-ordinator can send the marking grid and scenario to the examiner and the patient. This gives the examiners and patients a chance to familiarise themselves with the scenario and to ensure they are up to date with the clinical skills and techniques taught at the university. In this mailing clear details of where and when the examiner and patient are required can be included, along with maps of the university campus and the allocated building.

### The day before the OSCE

If possible, try to set up the OSCE environment (a clinical skills laboratory is commonly used) the day before the event is due to take place. Each station requires enough space for the student to examine or interview the patient. The examiners may require a table, and each examiner, patient and student will require a chair. Screens can be used to ensure that each station is separate from the other and the stations must not be so close that participants can be easily overheard. The stations must be clearly labelled with the station number and, if necessary, the type of station. If a bed or a couch is required, it must be available and be in safe working order. If a bed or examination couch is required, ensure that the bed linen is clean and there are enough pillows and a blanket to cover the patient. Each station will require spare paper and pens for the student to use if required. The OSCE co-ordinator must ensure that any diagnostic equipment required is in good working order and that they have spare batteries to hand in case they are needed (for example, to be used in an otoscope or ophthalmoscope).

The OSCE co-ordinator must ensure that each station has the following in a pack for the OSCE examiner and patient:
- the timetable for the day, including breaks and the post-session feedback meeting
- a list of participating students
- a complete station scenario with all instructions
- enough mark sheets, with a couple of spares
- the patient scenario
- the student instructions, including separate ones for students with special needs, such as dyslexia, who may require the student instructions in a larger font, or on coloured paper

- any pictures, laboratory results or additional information should be laminated if possible, as this deters the students from writing on them or taking them away when they leave the station.

## On the day of an OSCE session

### OSCE co-ordinator

The OSCE co-ordinators should make sure they arrive early at the OSCE venue. They should meet and greet the examiners, explain the set-up and go through the marking criteria and OSCE scenarios to ensure the examiners are happy with their roles. The examiners and patients can be asked to run through the scenario to ensure that all the marking criteria are correct and that the patient knows what to expect from the student. The OSCE co-ordinator should have overall responsibility for the smooth running of the day, ensuring that the OSCE session runs on schedule (this may include timing stations; if so, a timing device will be required) and checking that all participants are aware of their respective roles.

### Examiners and patients

Most OSCEs are run with simulated patient scenarios and will have two examiners at each station. One examiner observes and assesses the student's performance against the pre-determined marking criteria. The other examiner plays the patient role. In some universities, the person role-playing the patient is an actor who has been specifically trained to undertake OSCE scenarios. Some universities now use drama students to role-play patients in an OSCE as they are less expensive to employ. The clinical examiners may come from a pool of advanced nursing graduates who have undertaken OSCEs themselves and have attended an OSCE examiners workshop. Alternatively, they might be sourced from a network of academic colleagues. Some universities may also use medical doctors, such as general practitioners, as OSCE examiners, depending on their local clinical links and networks. All examiners and simulated patients should be familiar with the requirements of the OSCE assessment.

On the day of an OSCE session, if a station requires a physical examination, then the examiner should perform the requisite physical examination on the patient in order to identify any abnormalities that may be present. For example, if the station requires an examination of the ear, the examiner must know what the patient's tympanic membrane looks like, and if cerumen is present, then the examiner should expect students to comment on its presence during their individual examinations.

### Students

The role of the OSCE co-ordinator is to keep the students as calm as possible on the day. They will be nervous and may need help to relax before they start their OSCE. The co-ordinator should explain the OSCE procedure clearly to the students and ensure that they all understand what is practically expected of them during the OSCE. The respective roles of the examiner and patient should be explained clearly to the students. If the students are following a circuit where their start stations are all different, the OSCE co-ordinator needs to ensure that each student is clear about where they should start and the direction of the planned station circuit. If the students finish the station before the allocated time, then they should be advised to stay at the station and mentally recap the scenario, as they may suddenly remember an item they previously omitted. Ideally, the students should not leave a station until they are sure they have completed everything or else when their allocated station time has expired. In between stations, while an OSCE session is in progress students should be discouraged from discussing the OSCE station scenarios with each other, as the information that they convey to each other may not always be correct and potentially incorrect information could hamper the students' performances in other stations.

### OSCE external examiner/moderator

We believe that it is good practice to appoint an external examiner to critically evaluate each OSCE session to ensure consistency and equity of assessment across all the students. This person could be the external examiner responsible for assessing the traditional written components of assessment for a course, or they could be specially selected to critically appraise the OSCE assessment process. The OSCE external examiner should be familiar with advanced nursing practice and should have had recent experience of OSCE examining. The OSCE external examiner can also play a part in OSCE marking, as discussed later in chapter 10.

### At the end of the OSCE session

The OSCE co-ordinator may wish to convene a feedback session at the end of the OSCE session. Here the examiners and patients can report on how well their stations ran and whether or not, in their opinion, any changes to the stations should be made. This feedback session also gives the examiners and patients the opportunity to highlight to the academic team any perceived procedural difficulties the students may have encountered during the OSCE. This type of group feedback contributes to the face validity of individual OSCE stations. The end of the OSCE meeting can also be used as an opportunity for the examiners to give immediate appraisals of individual student performances; particularly for those students who gave cause for concern, or those who put in an outstanding performance. These immediate comments can then be used by the academic team to inform the OSCE marking process. A final and important activity for the co-ordinator is to collate all the students' exam papers and ensure they are ready for marking.

## OSCE examiner workshops

We have previously mentioned the use of OSCE workshops to support student learning. A useful adjunct to these student-focused workshops is to provide OSCE examiner-focused workshops. In our university all OSCE examiners are required to attend a preparatory OSCE examiners' workshop before being considered competent to undertake the role of an OSCE examiner. This ensures that all the examiners have been prepared to the same standard and fully understand their role.

The OSCE examiners' workshop is led by an academic who is responsible for running the OSCE in the advanced nursing programme. OSCE examiner workshops lasting for one day are offered by the university on a regular basis, once or twice every academic year. To encourage attendance potential participants can be made aware that attendance at a workshop can be cited as evidence of continuing professional development.

### Suggested format for an OSCE examiners' workshop

- Introduction to the programme of advanced nursing study being assessed by the OSCE.
- Defining the OSCE process; what is an OSCE?
- Validity and reliability of the OSCE.
- Number and type of OSCE stations being used.
- Length of each OSCE station.
- The range of advanced clinical skills being examined.
- From an overall perspective, what is being examined? For example, on a nurse practitioner programme the examination tests a range of key clinical skills to discern whether the nurse practitioner student can independently assess, plan, deliver and evaluate the advanced care of presenting patients.
- An introduction to student preparation for the OSCE.
- The criteria for becoming an OSCE examiner.
- The role of the OSCE examiner.
- Scoring the OSCE.

- Pass and referral criteria for OSCE stations.
- Practising OSCE examining and patient simulation in small groups of two to three participants, either with previously validated OSCE stations or with newly developed stations that require piloting.

### Suggested criteria for becoming an advanced nursing OSCE examiner

Potential OSCE examiners should:
- have graduated from the advanced nursing programme the OSCE seeks to assess (this requirement implies that the potential examiner will have also had experience of being an OSCE student)
- be experienced advanced nurses working within a relevant area of clinical practice, so that they that have the appropriate experience in the clinical area that they are required to examine
- have attended an OSCE examiners' workshop
- be able and willing to commit themselves to examining students.

### The role of the OSCE examiner

The role of the OSCE examiner at an individual OSCE station is to:
- observe the performance of the student at a particular clinical skill
- score the student performance according to the marking criteria
- ensure that the mark sheet is completed and has been checked for consistency, and that each criterion is complete
- contribute to the good conduct of the examination
- ensure that the students they examine have an equitable and consistent experience at the particular OSCE station for which they are responsible.

It is not the role of the OSCE examiner to:
- deviate from the marking criteria and ask the student questions that are not covered in the exam paper
- rewrite the station as they conduct the examination
- interfere with the patient role
- design their own scoring scheme
- teach the student during the examination. They assess only students' current knowledge and application of applied clinical skills.

Examiners should be made aware of their role function as detailed above during their OSCE examiner workshop.

**Summary activities for academic staff OSCE preparation**

○ Organise student and examiner preparation via workshops.

○ Plan the date, time and location of an OSCE session well in advance of an actual session.

○ Recruit examiners and patients for the OSCE session and reconfirm their attendance before the OSCE session.

○ Liaise with academic team members to decide on the selection of OSCE stations to be used.

○ Arrange for the printing of the OSCE exam papers.

○ If possible, set up the OSCE stations the day before.

○ Check in the examiners, patients and students.

○ Brief all the above parties on their respective roles.

○ Keep the OSCE session on schedule and ensure the OSCE stations are correctly timed.

○ Collate all the exam papers at the end of the OSCE session, and if a post-OSCE meeting is used, chair it and make notes of the examiners' comments.

## References

1 Pendleton D, Schofield T, Tate P, Havelock P. *The Consultation: an approach to learning and teaching.* Oxford: Oxford University Press; 1984.

2 Pendleton D, Schofield T, Tate P, Havelock P. *The New Consultation: developing doctor-patient communication.* Oxford: Oxford University Press; 2003.

3 Heath C, Luff P, Sanchez Svensson M. Video and qualitative research: analysing medical practice and interaction. *Med Educ.* 2007; 41: 109–16.

4 Corbally M. Considering video production? Lessons learned from the production of a blood pressure measurement video. *Nurse Educ Pract.* 2005; 5: 375–9.

5 Corbally, op. cit

6 Simulated OSCEs. Available at http://www.youtube.com/LSBUOSCE (accessed 9 Oct 2008)

# 4

# History taking OSCE stations

## What are history taking OSCE stations?

Typically, history taking OSCE stations seek to assess your ability to obtain an episodic or problem-focused history from a patient presenting with a specific common complaint, such as a cough, chest pain or urinary symptoms. It is possible that at the end of a history taking station, you will be asked to give a list of possible differential diagnoses relevant to the scenario. It is your ability to elicit accurate and detailed information from a patient within a structured analytical framework which is the underlying theme that will be assessed during the history taking OSCE. Taking a history from a patient is the fundamental feature of a consultation. Without accurate and analytical history taking it is impossible to establish a differential diagnosis for a patient's presenting problem. History taking formats utilise a structured framework for acquiring and organising health information about an individual patient. It is the focal point of the assessment process as it establishes the interactions and subsequent social relationship between nurse practitioner and patient; as such it is important that the style and tone of your history taking is responsive to the particular needs of an individual patient.

## Key activities and focused questions to ask in a history taking station

There are a number of key activities and focused questions that must be undertaken during a history taking station regardless of the scenario. These activities and questions are presented in sequence below and are also summarised on the following page:

## Key history taking activities

1  introducing yourself to the patient
2  asking initial questions
3  asking about the duration of the problem
4  asking if others have the same problem
5  asking about the severity/character of the problem
6  asking about the location/radiation of the problem
7  asking about the patient's self-help therapeutics
8  asking about the length of illness
9  asking about the associated symptoms
10  asking about the patient's perceptions

### 1 Introducing yourself to the patient

This will enable you to establish who the examiner is and who the patient is. Ensure that you sit down next to the patient or close to the patient and that you address the questions to the patient not to the examiner. This will demonstrate to the examiner that you are focusing on the patient. Remember that your body language is important and that you need to make sure the patient feels comfortable with you. If you are too far way and patient will feel that you are not connecting with them, and if you are too close they may feel inhibited by your presence.

### 2 Asking initial questions

Once you have introduced yourself, start your history inquiry with an open question, such as: 'How can I help you today?' or 'What brings you here today?' This type of open question will enable you to quickly establish the presenting problem, and therefore the scenario context of the particular history taking station. Try to listen to the patient's response without interruption. You may be yearning to ask the questions you have revised, but without listening carefully you may miss vital information. Once the patient has stopped speaking you can begin to clarify and expand the patient's story. While the open-ended question allows patients to tell you in their own words what they have come to see you for, please remember that they may not be as forthcoming with information as patients in normal clinical practice would be. It is up to you to demonstrate your ability to elicit information from patients by asking careful and structured questions. Continue to listen carefully to what the patient says to you, and if you need to, repeat and summarise what the patient has told you. This technique allows you to demonstrate that you have heard and understood what the patient has said, while giving you thinking time to formulate subsequent questions.

Having established the main presenting problem you need to find out more about its precise nature. Guide the patient to expand on potentially significant features of their chief complaint(s) and/or symptoms. The nature of their symptoms must be clarified, including their context, associations and chronology. You should always use language that is understandable by the patient.

Here you could use a mnemonic history taking device, such as 'OPQRSTU' to guide your questions, and to demonstrate to the examiner that you are able to coherently structure your history taking through careful consideration of the characteristics of the patient's presenting problem.

### Mnemonic history taking device

**O** – other people affected/other symptoms?
**P** – provocative and palliative?
**Q** – quality and quantity?
**R** – region, radiation and recurrence?
**S** – severity of symptoms/other symptoms?
**T** – timing and treatment?
**U** – what do *you* think is wrong (i.e. what the does the patient/carer think)?

Consolidate your initial question and develop the patient's response with these detailed follow-up questions that will help you further analyse the patient's problem(s):

### 3 Asking about the duration of the problem

Ask the patient exactly how long they have had their symptoms for. If they respond vaguely, such as 'for a few days', ask them to specify what they mean by 'few days'. Ask if they have ever had anything like this before? If so, are the symptoms presenting in the same way?

### 4 Asking about others with the same problem

Ask if anyone else in close contact with the patient, such as at home or work, have recently experienced similar symptoms. This question may enable you to establish whether or not the presenting problem could be an infectious illness, particularly if close contacts have been recently affected with similar symptoms.

### 5 Asking about the severity/character of the problem

Here you need to determine the severity of the symptoms. Ask the patient if the problem has affected their ability to perform their normal everyday activities, such as going to work. Has the problem affected their sleep? If the problem is causing pain or dysfunction you could use a rating scale of 1–10 to ask the patient how they would rate the severity of the pain or dysfunction.

Once you have ascertained the severity of the pain or problem, you must determine the precise nature of the pain or problem. Ask the patient to describe the pain or problem to you. For example, is it constant or intermittent? Does it occur only with certain activities, such as movement? What is the pain like? Is it stabbing, throbbing, cramp-like, or a dull ache? Does anything make the symptoms or pain worse, such as sleeping, being in one position, or walking? Does anything make the symptoms or pain better? If the patient is experiencing shortness of breath, ask how far they can walk before they have to stop and catch their breath.

These types of questions will help you to put the severity of the problem into perspective. If the problem is preventing the patient from performing normal activities such as working, dressing or bathing, then they will perceive the problem as being more serious than they will if they can still perform normal activities, and you should also take account of the potential seriousness and severity of the problem.

### 6 Asking about the location/radiation

Ask the patient the exact location of the problem. Is the symptom located in the same place or does it radiate anywhere else? If the patient is complaining of pain, ask them to point to where the pain is. Patients' perception of their anatomy is not always correct, but by asking them to point you can approximate the location of the problem.

### 7 Asking about the patient's self-help therapeutics

Try to establish what the patient has done to help themselves. This will also help you to understand the patient's own health beliefs in relation to the symptoms they are experiencing. For example, the following questions can help determine the patient's views on the use of analgesics or alternative medicines. Ask the patient if they have tried anything to relieve the symptoms? If so, what have they tried? How often have they been using the medicine or product? How much of the medicine or product have they used? Has it helped? How long did the relief last? When did they last take or use the medicine or product?

### 8 Asking about the length of the illness

Ask the patient if the symptoms are getting better, worse or staying the same. If they are changing, how are they changing and at what pace? Has a recent change in the symptoms prompted the patient's attendance? The life cycle of some disease processes are quite specific and therefore it is important to work out if the symptoms follow a recognised pattern or not. A common example of the involution of a disease would be the typical prodromal features of herpes zoster followed by the development of vesicular rash a few days later.

### 9 Asking about associated symptoms

Ask if they have noticed any other symptoms or problems since their present symptoms developed. These may or may not be related, but the question must be asked. Apart from generally asking about other symptoms you need to ask specific questions about particular other symptoms that may indicate certain problems. For example, in a patient with a suspected urinary tract infection you need to ask about back pain, nausea, vomiting, unusual vaginal discharge and vulval irritation, spots or sores. It is not be sufficient just to say 'do you have any other symptoms?' The patient may not volunteer information because they may not realise that a symptom could be related to the presenting problem, and their lack of this recognition can easily be part of an OSCE scenario.

### 10 Asking about the patient's perceptions

Questions here relate to determining the patient's ideas and concerns about their problem and their expectations for treatment. Ask the patient what they think the problem might be. What is the patient worried about in relation to their symptoms and why have they come to be seen today? What do they want to do about their presenting problem? Patients may have specific concerns related to their symptoms and this may be alarming them. It is important to find out about these concerns in order to directly respond to the needs of your patient. In patients presenting with a carer such as a child's parent, for example, they would also need to be included in this discussion.

At this point you will by now know a lot about the patient's presenting problem, and your problem-focused history taking may be coming to natural conclusion. This is an indication that it is time for you to ask some background questions from the patient.

## Background questions to ask in a history taking station
### Past medical history

We all know that in real life many patients are reluctant to reveal their medical history as they may think that any medical problems that they have had in the past are not relevant to their presenting complaint. This may well be the case, but it may not be, and it is up to you to make the distinction through an informed interpretation of the patient's medical history. The same provisos apply equally to OSCE patients; therefore you need to ask some specific questions about their past medical history. For example, ask the patient if they have any current ongoing medical problems. Also ask if they have ever been in hospital or had any operations, or been on long-term drug therapy. Using these types of focused questions may help you to obtain a more complete picture of the patient's past medical history.

### Family history

Once you have obtained the past medical history ask the patient if they have any family history that you may need to know about. Here you are searching for heritable disease amongst first- or second-degree relatives, such as siblings, parents and grandparents. Most commonly these include heart disease, diabetes and some forms of cancer. If there are any, then ask the patient to be as specific as possible. For example, if a parent died of a heart attack aged 45 years, this is more significant than a heart attack at 75 years of age.

### Medications/medication history

Now you can consider the medication history. Ask the patient if they are currently taking any prescribed medications. If the answer is yes, ask what medicine or medicines they take, what they are for, and the dose and frequency. People may be prescribed medicines but they may not take them as directed, so ask about their compliance with their prescribed medicines schedules. If they are not compliant, ask why they are not. Also ask if they have ever taken prescribed medicines for a period of time longer than a few days.

Following prescribed medicines move onto over-the-counter medicines. Ask if the patient is taking any medicines bought over the counter. If so, ask what the medicine is and how and when they are taking it. Also ask about the use of any herbal medicines, homeopathy, or other complementary alternative medicines or therapies.

### Allergies

Here you should be primarily concerned with any adverse reactions to medicines the patient has previously taken. If an adverse reaction occurred, was it a serious problem, such as anaphylaxis, requiring hospital treatment? Here you are trying to establish if there has been an anaphylactic reaction to a drug or a less serious adverse effect, such as an itchy rash. You may sometimes also need to ask the patient if they have experienced allergic reactions to non-medicinal products such as chemicals, food or latex.

### Social history

This part of the history taking may be sensitive for the patient or carer. Dependent on the OSCE station scenario, remember that you will be assessed on how you ask these types of socially orientated questions. If you practise asking lifestyle questions you will be more comfortable when you have to ask them. Try to remember that you are not being judgmental, but merely identifying risk factors for specific disease processes. Areas to cover in the social history are listed below.

*Occupation.* Ask about the patient's occupation and how long they have been employed in this job. Ask if they enjoy their work, as occupational unhappiness may be an underlying cause of stress or anxiety in the patient's presentation. Ask retired patients if they have ever worked. What did they do and how long did they work for? Also think about occupational environmental factors that may have an effect on the patient's presenting problem.

The occupation may give you a clue to establishing a differential diagnosis, as the presenting problem may be related to the occupation. If you are considering a mental health problem such as depression, occupation or occupational history may be significant.

*Social situation.* Ask who the patient is living with; on their own, with a spouse/partner, or with relatives or friends. Ask if they have any dependent children. What is their housing like? Is it suitable for them at the moment? If relevant to the patient's presentation ask if they have stairs to climb. Where is their bathroom? Do they have an easily accessible toilet?

These socially orientated questions will help to clarify the patient's social and occupational situation and may influence your management plan and help you to decide what to do next for your patient.

### Lifestyle questions

The following topics give insight into the patient's lifestyle, which may have a significant influence on a patient's presenting problem.

*Smoking.* The patient's smoking history may have a direct influence on the patient's presenting problem. Ask if they smoke. If so, what do they smoke, and how many per day? Ask for how long they have been smoking. If they say they do not smoke, ask if they have ever smoked and if so, when did they give up. What did they smoke and how many did they smoke a day? How long did they smoke for? With older people, it may also be useful to establish whether or not they were subjected to passive smoking, as this may also be a contributing factor in chronic illness.

*Alcohol.* As with smoking, alcohol consumption may also have a direct influence on the patient's presenting problem. Ask the patient if they drink alcohol; if so, how much per day/week? What sort of alcohol do they typically drink? If necessary ask the patient if they are aware of the recommended weekly safe alcohol limit for their gender.

*Recreational drugs.* Usage of recreational drugs may not always be relevant, but sometimes knowledge of their usage is required. This is a sensitive question and you may need to remind the patient of the confidentiality of their history. Ask the patient if they take any recreational drugs. If so, what drugs, when and how often do they typically use them. If they reply that they do not take recreational drugs, ask if they have ever taken them and, if so, how frequently. When did they last take them? What did they take?

*Foreign travel.* Travelling is common, but not everyone will have the recommended immunisations for specific countries. Consideration must be given to the risk of infectious tropical diseases. Ask the patient if they have had any recent foreign travel; if so, where? Ask if it was to a malarial area? Did they take any recommended malaria prophylaxis?

*Exercise/physical activity.* Ask the patient how physically active they are on an everyday basis. Do they undertake any exercise or sports activities? If so, what physical activity and how often?

## Gynaecological history (if appropriate)

Gynaecological questions are often indicated in female patients for many presenting problems. In women of childbearing age a key area to address is the patient's perceived risk of pregnancy, which is particularly important in women presenting with abdominal, pelvic or genito-urinary problems; especially to exclude the risk of ectopic pregnancy. Ask the patient if they think there is any chance they could be pregnant. Ask what form of contraception, if any, they use and if they have had any recent problems with this method.

Ask also when their last menstrual period was. Was it as normal? What is the normal length of their menstrual cycle? Is it regular? Ask if they have ever been pregnant. If so, how many times? What was the outcome of each pregnancy: full-term delivery, premature delivery, spontaneous abortion or therapeutic abortion? If relevant, enquire about their age of menarche or menopause, as appropriate. Also ask about the date of their last cervical smear and its results.

## Sexual health history

In some presentations the patient's sexual health history may be of relevance. Ask the patient if they are sexually active. Do they have a regular partner? Have they had any new sexual contacts in the 3 months prior to their presentation? When was their last sexual health screen? Have they ever had a sexually transmitted infection? If so, what sort and how long ago? How was it treated?

### ⫸❶⫸ Red flag questions

A key concept to consider in a patient's history is that of red flag questions (sometimes also called alarm symptoms). Red flags are crucial signs and symptoms that may indicate serious pathology in the context of the patient's chief complaint. For example, in a patient presenting with a cough it is essential to establish whether they have had haemoptysis, persistent fever, chest pain, persisting or worsening dyspnoea, or unintended weight loss as positive answers to any of these questions may potentially indicate serious problems such as a pneumonia, tuberculosis or lung cancer. In order to elicit any red flag symptoms it is important to ask the patient direct, easily understandable questions. For example, for the red flag of haemoptysis you should specifically ask the patient if they have coughed up any blood, rather than just asking if they have coughed anything up.

## Examples of specific question topics to cover in relation to different body systems

(These questions should be applied flexibly in conjunction with the previously presented history information)

### Respiratory history taking

The typical OSCE history taking scenario here is a patient presenting with a cough or shortness of breath.

- Biographical details – think about the age of your patient. For example, chronic obstructive pulmonary disease typically occurs in older people.
- Presenting symptoms.
- Current medical status: are they normally fit and well, or do they have a diagnosed medical condition?
- Past medical history of respiratory conditions, particularly asthma or chronic obstructive pulmonary disease: if present, how well is the condition normally controlled, what are the trigger factors, what respiratory-related medications do they take? What effect have these medications had? Has the condition required any hospital in-patient treatment?
- Family history – particularly respiratory conditions.
- Social history – housing, occupation, past occupations.

- Lifestyle – smoking, alcohol, recreational drugs, travel, exercise/physical activity.
- Medications – what type, prescribed, over the counter, herbal/alternative, when taken, how taken (think about compliance).
- Allergies (atopy is important here if there is a corresponding history of asthma).
- Recently in contact with anyone who has an infectious disease?
- Immunisations up to date (for children)?
- Presenting symptoms – duration of symptoms, when better, when worse, breathing pattern.
- Symptoms affecting sleep?
- Cough – type, is it productive? If so, what is the sputum like?

### ▶●▶  Red flags

- Have they coughed up any blood? Is there any blood-stained sputum? If so, what is that like?
- Is there any accompanying fever? If so, is it controlled on any antipyretic medication?
- Have there been any night sweats?
- Has there been any unintentional weight loss?

**TABLE 4.1** Marking criteria for history taking OSCE – respiratory/cough

| MARKING CRITERIA – RESPIRATORY COUGH |
| --- |
| Student introduces self and displays a open and warm approach to the patient |
| Student demonstrates a structured approach to history taking |
| Student uses open questions |
| Student establishes reason for patient attendance, and notes timing and onset of problem |
| Student asks about the nature of the patient's cough |
| Student asks about other symptoms such as ear, nose, and throat symptoms |
| Student elicits red flags<br>• haemoptysis<br>• fever<br>• chest pain<br>• breathlessness<br>• night sweats<br>• unintended weight loss |
| Student elicits past history of chest problems, general past medical history, drug history, allergies, smoking/alcohol consumption, and also social and travel history |
| Student elicits the patient's perspective of the problem |

## Ear, nose, throat and lymph node problems

A typical ear, nose and throat history scenario could be a patient presenting with a sore throat, sinus pain, or an earache.

Ears history: elicit:

- the onset of problem
- whether it was acute or gradual
- the severity of the pain (use a pain scale if necessary)
- whether the pain radiates anywhere else
- whether there is any ear discharge
- whether there is any bleeding from the ear
- whether any analgesia is used
- whether there is any past medical history of ear problems, such as infection, grommets or ear wax
- whether there is any recent upper respiratory tract infection symptoms
- whether there is any hearing loss
- whether there is any tinnitus
- whether there is any vertigo or dizziness
- whether the patient has been exposed to occupational environmental noise
- whether the patient has used cotton buds to clean the ears
- whether the patient has any experience of recent ear trauma? This would include acoustic trauma
- whether there is any history of a foreign body in the ear
- whether the patient has been swimming/diving recently
- whether the patient had any recent any air travel
- whether the patient uses earphones regularly.

If the patient complains of hearing loss, ask:

- Was the hearing loss gradual or sudden?
- Is it partial or complete?
- Is it in both ears?
- Is there any history of ear wax problems?
- Is there any history of a foreign body in the ear?
- Is there a family history of hearing loss?
- Have you had any surgery or trauma to their ears?
- Have you had any serious systemic illness?
- Are you taking any potentially ototoxic drugs?
- Have you had any exposure to loud noise (acoustic trauma)?
- Have you had any associated vertigo (sensation of spinning) or dizziness?

Nose
- Is there nasal discharge? If so, what colour?
- Have you had any nose bleeds?
- Does your nose feel blocked?
- If so, is it constant or only in the day/night?
- Is the problem related to the seasons?
- What aggravates the problem?
- Have you taken any medicines to relieve the congestion?
- How effective was the medication?
- Do you suffer with frequent head colds?
- Do you have any sinus pain?
- If so, is it over your forehead or face?
- Have you had any recent injury to the face or nose?
- Do you have a history of nose bleeds?
- Do you have any allergies?
- Has your sense of smell altered in any way?
- Do you use or have you ever used inhaled drugs, such as medicinal nasal sprays or recreational drugs?
- Have you had any previous nose surgery?

Mouth
- Do you have a history of mouth sores or lesions?
- Do you have toothache (possible cause of referred pain)?
- Do you have bleeding gums?
- Do you go to the dentist regularly?
- Do you any voice hoarseness?
- Do you have any pain or difficulty in swallowing?
- Do you have any altered taste sensations, if so, what?

Throat
- Do you have a history of a sore throat?
- When did your symptoms start?
- Have you taken any analgesics?
- How effective has the analgesia been?
- Is there any associated fever?
- Are you able to swallow?
- Have you started on any recent new medications?

Lymph nodes
- Was the onset of symptoms acute or gradual?

- Do you have any tender swellings, lumps, nodules in your neck?
- Have you noted any swellings or lumps elsewhere on your body? (Common areas would be the axillae or groin).
- How long have they been there?
- Are they painful?
- How severe is the pain? (Use a pain-rating scale.)
- Do you have any associated thyroid problems? For example weight changes, thinning hair, lethargy.
- Do you have a cough?
- Do you have any mouth or throat problems?
- How do you feel otherwise? For example, have you been able to maintain your normal everyday activities?

### ➤❶➤ Red flags

- Have the swellings changed in size?
- Have you had any fever?
- Have you had any night sweats?
- Have you had any unintentional weight loss?

**TABLE 4.2** Marking criteria for history taking OSCE – ENT

| MARKING CRITERIA – SORE THROAT |
| --- |
| Student introduces self |
| Student displays open and warm approach to the patient |
| Student demonstrates a structured approach to history taking |
| Student uses open questions |
| Student establishes reason for patient attendance |
| Student asks about any other ear, nose and throat symptoms |
| Student asks where the pain is located and if it radiates |
| Student asks when the pain started |
| Student asks if the pain is constant or intermittent |
| Student asks the patient to describe the pain using a severity scale 1–10 |
| Student asks if there have been any preceding symptoms of a cold, sore throat or temperature |
| Student asks if anything makes the pain better |
| Student asks if anything makes the pain worse |
| Student asks if the pain disturbs the patient's sleep or prevents any normal activities of daily living? |
| Student asks if the patient has any symptoms of vertigo or dizziness |

(continued)

---

**MARKING CRITERIA – SORE THROAT**

---

Student asks if the patient has any abnormal noises in their ear

Student asks if the patient has any hearing impairment

Student asks if there is a risk of a foreign body in the ear

Student asks if there is any history of trauma to the ear (physical or acoustic)?

Student asks if there is any discharge from ear

Student asks if there is any bleeding from ear

Student asks if the patient has recently been swimming/diving

Student asks about recent air travel

Student asks about the patient's medication for this problem and its effect

Student asks about the patient's drug history

Student asks about the patient's allergies

Student asks about the patient's related medical history, e.g. previous problems with ears

Student asks about the patient's past medical history

Student asks about the patient's family history

Student asks about the patient's social history

Student asks about the patient's history of smoking

Student asks about the patient's use of alcohol

Student asks about the patient's use of recreational drugs

Student asks about the patient's exercise

Student elicits the patient's perception of the problem

## Key questions for patients presenting with an eye problem

A typical scenario here would be a person presenting with an acute red eye, with or without accompanying pain.

- How long ago did the problem start?
- Was the onset of the symptoms acute or gradual?
- Have there been any changes in your vision, for example, blurring, blind spots, distorted straight lines, floaters/stars?
- Do you have any double vision (diplopia)?
- Do you have any actual eye pain?
- Do you have any periorbital pain?
- Assess the severity of the pain. (Use a pain-rating scale.)
- Is there any redness of the eye?
- Is there swelling?
- Is there any itching of the eye?
- Is there any discharge – if so, what sort? Is it watery or purulent? If

purulent, are the lids stuck together on waking? What colour is the purulent discharge?

- Do you use glasses?
- Do you use contact lenses?
- How do you care for your contact lenses?
- Has there been any recent trauma to the eyes?
- Is there any recent history of a foreign body in the eye?

Past medical history
- Do you any history of eye problems?

Family history
- Is there any family history of eye disease such as glaucoma?

Medication history
- Have you recently used topical eye medicines, including over-the-counter and prescribed products.

**TABLE 4.3** Marking criteria for history taking OSCE – red eye

| MARKING CRITERIA –RED EYE |
| --- |
| Student introduces self |
| Student displays open and warm approach to the patient |
| Student demonstrates a structured approach to history taking |
| Student uses open questions |
| Student establishes reason for patient attendance |
| Student asks the patient about any other symptoms/otherwise unwell |
| Student asks re: pain location/radiation |
| Student asks when the pain started |
| Student asks if the pain constant or intermittent |
| Student asks the patient to describe the pain using a severity scale 1–10 |
| Student asks if there have been any preceding symptoms |
| Student asks if the patient has any eye pain |
| Student asks if there is a history of foreign body in the eye |
| Student asks if there is a history of trauma to the eye |
| Student asks if the patient wears contact lenses |
| Student asks if the patient is experiencing any visual disturbance (e.g. acuity, floaters, diplopia) |
| Student asks if the patient has noted any discharge from the eye |
| Student establishes the colour of the discharge |

*(continued)*

MARKING CRITERIA –RED EYE

Student asks if the patient has had crusted lids on waking

Student asks if the patient has noted any itching of the eye

Student asks if the patient has noted any eyelid swelling or pain

Student asks if the patient has noted any periorbital pain, redness, rashes or swelling

Student asks if they have any history of eye problems

Student asks about use of medication for any problem and its effect

Student asks if there is any of history of drugs

Student asks about allergies

Student asks about past medical history

Student asks about family history

Student asks about social history

Student asks about smoking

Student asks about alcohol use

Student elicits the patient's perception of the problem

## Key questions to ask a patient presenting with abdominal problems

Typical examples of abdominal related problems are a patient presenting with abdominal pain and urinary symptoms, or a patient presenting with a history of dyspepsia.

- How long ago did the problem start?
- Have you had any previous similar problems?
- Do you have any abdominal pain?
- Is the abdominal pain intermittent or constant?
- Was the onset of the pain acute or gradual?
- Please point to the location of pain.
- Please describe the character of the pain (aching, stabbing, throbbing).
- Is there any radiation of the pain?
- How severe is the pain? (Use a pain-rating scale, such as 1–10, or a visual analogue scale.)
- Does the pain disturb your sleep?
- Do you have any nausea and/or vomiting?
- Do you have any problems passing urine? Specifically have you noticed any dysuria, frequency, urgency or nocturia?
- (For men) Do you have or have you had any testicular pain, swelling or lumps, or any urethral discharge?
- (For women) Do you have or have you had an unusual vaginal discharge or any vaginal/vulval irritation, spots or sores. You may also need to ask

if they have experienced any dyspareunia (vaginal and/or pelvic) as this may indicate the presence of a vaginal or pelvic infection.

- If there are any positive responses to the above gender-specific questions you may also need to elicit a brief sexual health history by asking questions such as: Do you have a regular partner? Have you had any recent new sexual contacts (for example in the preceding six weeks)? Have you had any sexually transmitted infections before? When was your last sexual health screen?
- Have you noted any change in your bowel habits? Specifically, when were your bowels last open? Do you feel constipated? Have you had any recent diarrhoea? If there is a history of diarrhoea you may need to ask about their recent travel history.
- Do you have any change in appetite, such as a decreased appetite?
- Do you have any known food intolerance?
- Please tell me about your diet and diet history.
- Please tell me about your alcohol use and your history of alcohol use.
- Please tell me about your smoking and your smoking history.

### ►❶► Red flags
- Have you had any recent unintended weight loss? If yes, this often serious symptom requires further evaluation with the following supplementary questions.
- Has your appetite been maintained or has it increased or decreased recently?
- What is the specific time span for your weight loss?
- Has the weight loss affected your enjoyment of food?
- Please describe your normal daily eating pattern, including quantities and timing.
- Do you have any difficulty swallowing food or fluids (dysphagia)? If yes, this potentially serious symptom requires further evaluation with these types of questions.
- Where does the food get stuck?
- How long have you had the symptoms – days or weeks?
- Is the symptom intermittent or progressive? A gastro-oesophageal malignancy normally follows a short, rapidly progressing course.
- Has there been any regurgitation of food or fluids?

### ►❶► Other abdominal red flags
- Have you noticed any rectal bleeding?
- Have you vomited any blood or noted any blood-stained vomit?

- In women remember to ask specifically about the timing of their last menstrual period and their perceived risk of pregnancy.

## Key questions to ask a patient presenting with diarrhoea

A typical OSCE scenario here might be a patient returning from travel abroad who has recently developed diarrhoea.

- Please describe your normal stool frequency and consistency.
- How long have you had the diarrhoea for?
- What changes have occurred? For example, how many times per day do you have diarrhoea?
- What do you mean by diarrhoea?
- What is the consistency of your stools?
- What is the colour of your stools?
- What is the odour of your stools?
- Is there any associated abdominal pain with the diarrhoea? For example, abdominal cramps often immediately precede episodes of diarrhoea.
- Does the diarrhoea disturb your sleep? For example, do you have to get up in the night to open your bowels?
- Have any others in contact with you had similar problems?
- Can you possibly attribute the cause of the diarrhoea to any food you have eaten?
- Have you had associated nausea and vomiting?
- Has your appetite been affected? Have you been able to eat and/or drink?

### Red flags

- Is there any blood in the stool?
- Is there any mucus in the stool?
- Have you had any recent foreign travel? What countries have you visited? Did you adhere to food and water hygiene precautions?
- Have you had any recent unintended weight loss?

TABLE 4.4 Marking criteria for history taking OSCE – abdominal pain/dyspepsia

| MARKING CRITERIA – ABDOMINAL PAIN/DYSPEPSIA |
| --- |
| Student's general approach– introduction, explanation and warmth |
| Student elicits the patient's presenting problem |
| Student undertakes symptom analysis using a structured approach |
| Student asks when the problem started |
| Student asks about provoking factors – food, alcohol |

(continued)

| MARKING CRITERIA – ABDOMINAL PAIN/DYSPEPSIA |
| --- |
| Student asks about relieving factors – food, antacids |
| Student asks about quality of pain – sharp/dull |
| Student asks about quantity of pain – episodic, constant |
| Student asks about radiation of pain |
| Student asks about severity of pain |
| Student asks about the timing of the pain – at night/when asleep |
| Student asks about appetite – loss/increase/no change |
| Student asks about associated symptoms: nausea and vomiting |
| Student asks about vomiting of blood |
| Student asks about any bowel changes, including presence of blood |
| Student asks about any unintended weight loss |
| Student considers cardiac symptoms |
| Student elicits whether any other health problems/review of systems |
| Student asks about lifestyle: family status |
| Student asks about occupation |
| Student asks about diet |
| Student asks about smoking |
| Student asks about alcohol |
| Student asks about recreational drugs |
| Student asks about allergies |
| Student explores current stressors |
| Student explores family history |
| Student asks about past medical history |
| Student asks about current medication, including usage of over-the-counter medicines |
| Student elicits the patient's perception of the problem |

**TABLE 4.5** Marking criteria for history taking OSCE – abdominal pain/dysuria

| MARKING CRITERIA – ABDOMINAL PAIN/DYSURIA |
| --- |
| Student's general approach to patient: introduction, warmth and empathy |
| Student asks about asks open-ended questions demonstrating sensitivity and appropriate communication skills throughout |
| Student determines the patient's presenting complaint (abdominal pain and dysuria) |
| Student uses symptom analysis OPQRST framework |
| Student asks about other symptoms<br>• frequency<br>• urgency<br>• nocturia |

*(continued)*

## MARKING CRITERIA – ABDOMINAL PAIN/DYSURIA

Student asks about other symptoms (cont.)

- unusual vaginal discharge
- vaginal/vulval irritation, spots or sores

Student asks about provoking factors: does abdominal pain increase with micturition

Student asks about relieving factors: is abdominal pain partially relieved with paracetamol

Student asks about quality/quantity of abdominal pain and intermittent pain

Student asks about region/radiation: supra-pubic abdominal pain, no back pain

Student asks about recurrence: asks if patient has experienced similar problems in past

Student asks about severity of problem: uses a pain-rating scale to assess the severity of abdominal pain/dysuria, and its effect on the patient's life, e.g. time off work

Student asks about timing: how long ago did the abdominal pain start, duration of dysuria, duration of other urinary symptoms

**Red flags**: student asks about

- nausea and vomiting
- haematuria
- fever
- possibility of pregnancy and last menstrual period
- history of abdominal/back trauma
- weight loss

Student asks about lifestyle

- exercise
- occupation
- travel history

Student asks about

- past medical history
- any history of previous abdominal problems, such as cystitis

Student asks about drug history

Student asks if the patient has tried any over-the-counter medicines and their effect

Student asks about allergies

Student asks if the patient smokes or has ever smoked

Student asks about the patient's weekly alcohol intake

Student asks about the patient's sexual health history

- Does she currently have a partner?
- Has she had any new sexual contacts?
- When was her last sexual health screen?

Student explores the patient's perceptions of the problem

Student asks the patient what they would like to do about the problem

Student demonstrates a structured approach to focused history taking

## Key questions to ask a patient presenting with cardiovascular problems

OSCEs related to cardiovascular problems are popular choices as cardiovascular problems such as chest pain, breathlessness and palpitations are common and potentially serious presentations in practice.

General questions for patients presenting with cardiovascular problems
- Do you have any chest pain?
- Have you experienced any shortness of breath?
- Do you have a cough?
- Do you feel excessively tired?
- Do you have swollen ankles/feet?
- Have you noticed a change in skin colour?

Relevant past medical history of concern includes:
- previously identified cardiac disease/problems
- previous investigations for cardiac disease
- hypertension
- high cholesterol
- heart murmur
- rheumatic fever
- anaemia.

Relevant family history includes:
- cardiac disease
- hypertension
- diabetes.

Relevant lifestyle factors to enquire about includes:
- diet
- exercise
- smoking, including smoking history
- alcohol, including alcohol history.

Specific questions to ask a patient presenting with cardiovascular problems
Chest pain
- When does it occur – on exertion or at rest?
- Is the pain constant or intermittent?
- Where is the pain?/Can you point to where it is?
- Was the onset of the pain gradual or sudden?

- Does the pain radiate anywhere, for example, down an arm, or into the jaw?
- Does the pain occur after exercise?
- Is it worse after eating a large meal?
- How long do you have to wait until the pain subsides?
- Does anything relieve the pain, for example, rest or a change of position?
- Has there been any history of chest trauma or exercise or heavy lifting (this question reveals chest pain of a musculoskeletal origin as opposed to a cardiac cause).
- If you suspect musculoskeletal chest wall pain, ask the patient if they have an intermittent sharp pain which gets worse on coughing or sneezing, inspiration and movement.
- You may also need to explore any potential cough history in more detail, as per respiratory history taking.
- Do you use analgesia to relieve the pain? (This could include cardiac drugs such as glyceryl trinitrate, or simple analgesics such as paracetamol).

Additional questions for palpitations
- Does your heartbeat feel regular or irregular?
- How long do the palpitations last for?
- Do you have them at present?
- What were you doing before you experienced the palpitations?
- Have you experienced palpitations before? If yes, has this required any medical investigations or treatment?
- Are the palpitations accompanied by chest pain, dyspnoea or faintness?
- Have you recently experienced any stressful life events or do you feel anxious?
- Have you recently taken any recreational drugs? (Drugs such as cocaine or amphetamines can commonly cause palpitations).
- How much caffeine do you normally drink? (Excess caffeine is a further common cause of palpitations).

**TABLE 4.6** Marking criteria for history taking OSCE – cardiac chest pain

| MARKING CRITERIA – CHEST PAIN |
| --- |
| Student's general approach to patient (warmth, empathy, introduces self) |
| Student's approach is client-centred, uses open questions |
| Student uses a structured approach to history taking and exploring the nature of the problem |
| Student elicits provocative factors, e.g. what makes the pain worse? |

*(continued)*

45

### MARKING CRITERIA – CHEST PAIN

Student elicits palliative factors, e.g. did anything help the pain?

Student elicits quality of pain, e.g. can you describe the pain?

Student elicits quantity of pain, e.g. how long did it last for?

Student's asks about region and radiation, e.g. can you point to where the pain was? Did it travel anywhere?

Student elicits severity of pain (using a scale of 1–10)

Student elicits timing of pain, e.g. when did it happen?

Student elicits patient's past medical history

Student elicits patient's current medication

Student elicits patient's family history

Student elicits patient's social situation

Student elicits patient's smoking history

Student assesses other cardiovascular risk factors, e.g. alcohol intake

Student elicits patient's ideas/concerns

## Dyspnoea/shortness of breath

- Have you experienced shortness of breath?
- Do you currently feel breathless?
- When does it occur?
- How much can you do before becoming breathless?
- Do you wake up at night gasping for breath? If so, is it relieved by sitting up?
- How many pillows do you need to sleep?
- Have you noticed any wheezing?
- Do you have a cough? If so, is there any sputum, and what colour is it?
- Have you noticed that your ankles have become swollen?
- Do you have to get up in the night to pass urine?

**TABLE 4.7** Marking criteria for history taking OSCE – dyspnoea

### MARKING CRITERIA – DYSPNOEA

Student introduces self

Student has a warm approach to the patient

Student uses a structured approach to history taking

Student establishes the nature of the problem

Student elicits when the problem started

*(continued)*

MARKING CRITERIA – DYSPNOEA

Student elicits if any one else close to the patient has been ill with similar symptoms recently

Student elicits provoking factors, e.g. exercise, any recent respiratory tract infections

Student elicits relieving factors, e.g. rest

Student asks if the patient is wheezing

Student elicits the severity of the problem (may use a scale)

Student elicits if the problem affects the patient's activities of daily living

Student asks if the patient is experiencing any another associated problems

Student asks if the patient has a cough

Student establishes if the cough is productive – and the colour of sputum, e.g. green/yellow

Student asks if the patient has noticed any haemoptysis

Student asks if the patient has weight loss

Student asks if the patient has any changes in appetite

Student asks if the patient has ankle oedema

Student asks if the patient has orthopnea

Student asks about the patient's significant past medical history

Student asks about the patient's significant family history

Student asks about the patient's lifestyle: smoking habits

Student asks about the patient's use of alcohol

Student asks about the patient's exercise

Student asks about the patient's occupation

Student asks about the patient's home circumstances

Student asks about the patient's current use of medications

Student asks if the patient has any known allergies

Student asks about the patient's compliance with any medications

Student elicits patient's self-help to date

Student asks patient what they think is wrong

## Peripheral vascular system

- Do you get leg pain?
- Do you get leg cramp?
- Is the pain relieved by rest?
- How far can you walk before you experience the leg pain?
- Have you noticed any skin colour changes on your arms or legs?
- Have you noticed any loss of hair to the lower legs?
- Have you noticed any leg or ankle swelling?

**TABLE 4.8** Marking criteria for history taking OSCE – ischaemic leg pain

| MARKING CRITERIA – ISCHAEMIC LEG PAIN |
| --- |
| Student introduces self |
| Student conducts a patient-centred consultation, using open-ended questions |
| Student establishes patient's main problem |
| Student elicits provocative symptoms (exercise) |
| Student elicits palliative symptoms (rest) |
| Student elicits how far the patient can walk before the pain comes on |
| Student asks the patient to describe the pain |
| Student asks about the severity of the pain (using a pain scale) |
| Student asks if the pain radiates anywhere |
| Student asks about the timing of the pain |
| Student elicits the patient's past medical history |
| Student elicits the patient's current health status |
| Student elicits the patient's relevant family history |
| Student elicits the patient's current medication |
| Student asks about the patient's allergies |
| Student asks about the patient's smoking history |
| Student elicits whether the patient has noticed any changes in appearance of the legs or feet |
| Student elicits how this is affecting the patient's lifestyle |
| Student elicits if patient has tried any self-help remedies |
| Student elicits what the patient thinks the problem is |

## Key questions related to the neurological system

Possible OSCE scenarios here might be a patient presenting with a headache, dizziness, a transient ischaemic attack or cerebral vascular attack symptoms, or the assessment of a minor head injury.

### Brief tests for the assessment of cognitive function

Specially designed abbreviated mental tests or mini mental state exams which are routinely included in clinical examination textbooks[1,2] can be deployed to assess the cognitive function of OSCE patients presenting with possible signs of confusion or disorientation. These mental state tests typically give you a quick, yet objective assessment of a patient's cognitive function. Dependent on the format of your university's OSCEs, you would either need to revise and learn the sequence of a selected mental state test in order to use it in an OSCE station, or else you may be able to name a selected test that you could use, and you would then be given the score for your particular OSCE patient.

### Key questions to ask a patient presenting with a headache

- How long have you had the headache for?
- Please describe the headache to me.
- Please indicate where the headache is.
- Is the headache preceded by any aura-type sensations, such as flashing lights?
- How bad is the headache? (You could use a pain-rating scale.)
- Have you ever had a headache like this before?
- Do you have a history of headaches?
- Does the pain radiate to anywhere else?
- Is the headache intermittent or constant?
- Have you have taken anything to relieve the headache? If yes, ask how effective the analgesia was.
- Can you think of any precipitating factors that may have caused the headache, for example, dietary or environmental factors?

### ➤❶➤ Red flags

- Has the headache ever woken you from sleep?
- Is this the worst headache you have ever experienced?
- Do you have any neck stiffness?
- Do you have a fever?
- Have you experienced any visual disturbances?
- Have you noticed any facial numbness or tingling?
- Have you got any numbness or tingling anywhere else on your body?
- Have you had a recent head injury?
- Do you have any associated dizziness?
- (In women) Do you take the combined oral contraceptive pill (particularly of concern with a focal migraine)?
- Do you have a family history of headaches?

**TABLE 4.9** Marking criteria for history taking OSCE – headache

| MARKING CRITERIA – HEADACHE HISTORY |
| --- |
| Student Introduces self |
| Student displays a patient-centred communication style both verbally and non-verbally |
| Student identifies presenting problem, using open questioning |

(continued)

---

MARKING CRITERIA – HEADACHE HISTORY

---

Student asks about precipitating factors: red wine, stress

Student elicits quality of pain: asks patient to describe headache

Student elicits quantity of headaches, i.e., their frequency and changes in frequency

Student asks about their radiation/unilateral or bilateral

Student asks about their severity: using a pain scale

Student asks about their timing: during the day, at work and weekends

Student asks about their relief, e.g. sleeping in a dark room

Student asks about any associated symptoms: nausea, numbness, blurred vision, photophobia

**Student asks about red flag symptoms**: vomiting without nausea, sudden onset, thunderclap, waking the patient from sleep, collapse, fever

Student asks about the patient's self-help strategies, e.g. sleep, paracetamol

Student asks about the patient's past medical history

Student asks about the patient's family history of headaches

Student elicits the patient's social circumstances, including job and computer use

Student elicits the patient's current medication

Student elicits the patient's allergies

Student elicits the patient's smoking history

Student elicits the patient's alcohol history

Student elicits the patient's use of recreational drugs

Student elicits the patient's exercise habits

Student elicits the patient's dietary history

Student elicits the patient's health beliefs and concerns

---

## Key questions to ask a patient presenting with musculoskeletal problems

Typical OSCE scenarios that may be used for musculoskeletal problems are low back pain, shoulder pain and knee pain, as these are common presentations, but ones which often cause anxiety for students as they often feel less confident in assessing patients presenting with musculoskeletal problems. The presenting problems may be due to either acute minor injuries or alternatively acute or long-term inflammatory overuse conditions, such as tendonitis or arthritis. The distinction between injury and inflammation is important to determine and a key activity for assessing patients with musculoskeletal problems in an OSCE is to determine the exact nature of a patient's presenting problem(s) as it may not be initially clear from a patient's opening statement if they have either actually sustained an injury, or if they have an inflammatory overuse problem, or else an exacerbation of a long-term musculoskeletal condition. Establishing the type of musculoskeletal problem (i.e., is it an injury or an inflammatory condition?) from the outset of the OSCE will influence your clinical problem solving.

If an OSCE patient reports a history of musculoskeletal-type pain with no actual history of trauma reported in reply to your direct questioning their problem is most likely to be an acute inflammatory condition which has occurred as a result of musculoskeletal overuse in activities such as changed or increased exercise patterns, or repetitive exercise or movements. Establish from the patient what the underlying cause of potential inflammatory pain could be, as sometimes they may not tell you what caused the pain until you have elicited it in your history taking questions.

### General questions
- Has there been a history of trauma?
- Please specify exactly where the affected area is, and whether you have had a recent history of trauma?
- Can you describe the mechanism of the injury?
- What activities were you able to undertake immediately after the injury; for example, were you able to bear weight on the injured side, and have you been able to continue doing so?
- Is this a new problem or a chronic problem?
- Do you have any pain?
- What makes it better? What makes it worse? (Remember that musculoskeletal pain is typically a sharp pain which increases or occurs on movement).
- Have you taken anything to relieve the pain? How effective was it?
- How bad is the pain? (Use a pain-rating scale.)
- How has the pain affected your everyday activities?
- Is there any swelling in the affected area?
- Is there any stiffness in the joint?
- Is there any bruising?
- Does the joint feel hot to touch?
- Are there any limitations in the joint movement?
- Is there any pain or cramp in the muscles?
- Is there any muscular weakness?
- Do you have any associated neurological symptoms such as paraesthesia in the area distal to the site of inflammation or injury?

### Key questions to ask a patient presenting with lower back pain
- Has there been a history of trauma? If so, is it indirect (e.g. lifting/

exercise) or direct (e.g. a direct blow)? Consider referral to A&E if the trauma was direct.

- Do you have lower back pain?
- Have you ever had lower back pain before?
- Do you have any thoracic back pain? (This could be related to other problems such as cardiac or respiratory).
- Please indicate the location of your pain.
- What were you doing prior to experiencing the back pain?
- What provokes the pain?
- What relieves the pain?
- Have you taken any analgesics (such as over-the-counter paracetamol)?
- How effective was it?
- Please describe the pain.
- Is the pain in one place or does it radiate anywhere else?
- How severe is the pain? (Use a pain scale.)
- Is the pain intermittent or constant?
- Are there any associated symptoms, e.g. tenderness?

### ▶◑▶ Red flags

- Is there any leg muscle weakness?
- Is there any tingling in your legs or feet?
- Is there any sensation loss in your legs or feet?
- Is there any numbness in your perineal (saddle) area?
- Do you have any bowel problems, for example, an inability to open your bowels or incontinence?
- Do they have any urinary problems, for example, an inability to pass urine or incontinence? Do you have any dysuria, frequency or urgency (urinary tract infection)?

### Key questions to ask a patient presenting with shoulder pain

- Do you have a history of trauma?
- Do you have any neck pain?
- Where exactly is the shoulder pain located?
- What provokes the pain? Are there any particular shoulder or neck movements which cause the pain?
- What relieves the pain?
- Have you taken any analgesics (such as the over-the-counter paracetamol)?
- How effective was it?
- Please describe the pain.

- Is the pain in one place or does it radiate anywhere else?
- How severe is the pain? (Use a pain scale.)
- How has the shoulder pain affected your everyday life/physical activities?
- Is the pain intermittent or constant?
- Do you have any previous history of shoulder problems or shoulder surgery?

### ➤❗ Red flags

- Other potentially serious causes for shoulder pain include cardiac chest pain or referred pain from abdominal/pelvic pathologies.

### Key questions to ask a patient presenting with knee pain

- Do you have a history of trauma?
- Do you have any hip pain?
- Where exactly is the knee pain located?
- What provokes the pain? Are there any particular knee or hip movements which cause the pain?
- What relieves the pain?
- Have you taken any analgesics (such as the over-the-counter paracetamol)?
- How effective was it?
- Please describe the pain.
- Is the pain in one place or does it radiate anywhere else?
- How severe is the pain? (Use a pain scale.)
- How has the knee pain affected your everyday life or physical activities/ exercise?
- Is the pain intermittent or constant?
- Do you have a previous history of knee problems or knee surgery?

**TABLE 4.10** Marking criteria for history taking OSCE – back pain

| MARKING CRITERIA – BACK PAIN HISTORY |
| --- |
| Student's general approach to patient: introduction, warmth, and empathy |
| Student asks open-ended questions demonstrating sensitivity and appropriate communication skills throughout |
| Student determines the patient's presenting complaint (back pain) |
| Student does a symptom analysis using OPQRST framework<br>• asks about symptoms, such as urinary, pregnancy/last menstrual period<br>• asks about other provoking factors, e.g. movement<br>• asks about relieving factors, e.g. rest<br>• asks about quality/quantity of pain, e.g. sharp, dull, constant, episodic. |

*(continued)*

---

MARKING CRITERIA – BACK PAIN HISTORY

---

Student does a symptom analysis using OPQRST framework (cont.)

- asks if pain is localised or radiates
- asks about severity of pain, e.g. scale of 1–10 and/or effects on activities of daily living
- asks about timing – when the problem started and duration of the pain

**Red flags**: student asks about

- loss of bowel and/or bladder continence or urinary retention (altered bowel or bladder function)
- perineal numbness (saddle anaesthesia)

Student asks about symptoms related to musculoskeletal back pain

- altered lower limb sensations and/or numbness
- altered lower limb muscle strength and/or motor function

Student asks about the patient's lifestyle

- exercise
- occupation

Student asks about past medical history, including history of previous back problems

Student asks about any drug history

Student asks about any allergies

Student asks if any analgesic medicines tried and their effect

Student explores patient's perceptions of what the problem is

Student asks the patient what they would like to do about the problem

Student demonstrates a structured approach to focused history taking

---

## Skin complaint history taking

A typical OSCE history taking scenario here could be a patient presenting with an inflammatory skin condition such as eczema or psoriasis, or alternatively a vesicular, or petechial/purpuric rash.

- When did the problem start/what is the chronology of the presenting problem?
- Is it itchy?
- Is it painful?
- Is it red?
- Is there any discharge/exudate?
- Is it discrete or is it widespread?
- Is it unilateral or bilateral?
- Did it start in one specific area?
- Are you in contact with any other people with a similar problem?
- Do you have a past medical history of skin problems, such as allergies, eczema or psoriasis?
- Do you have a family history of skin problems?
- Are you using any new medications or have you changed medications?

- If you use any topical medications (including emollients) how compliant are you with them?
- Please describe your daily hygiene routine and say what soaps and cosmetics you use.
- Are there any occupational factors, such as usage of latex gloves or chemical exposure, that could be causing this?

### ▶◉▶ Red flags

- Do you have any associated illness symptoms?
- Do you feel unwell?
- Do you have any fever?
- If the patient does feel unwell or has a fever, consider asking about meningeal symptoms.
- Is there any unexplained bruising of the skin (i.e. petechial/purpuric rash)?

TABLE 4.11 Marking criteria for history taking OSCE – skin/eczema on hands

| MARKING CRITERIA – SKIN/ECZEMA ON HANDS |
| --- |
| Student introduces self to the patient |
| Student establishes a rapport with the patient |
| Student demonstrates structured history taking skills |
| Student asks open-ended questions |
| Student elicits provocative factors |
| Student elicits palliative factors |
| Student elicits quality of symptoms |
| Student elicits region of symptoms |
| Student elicits radiation of symptoms (skin areas affected) |
| Student elicits severity of symptoms (including possible signs of superficial infection) |
| Student elicits timing of symptoms |
| Student elicits any other associated symptoms |
| Student elicits further information about any allergies |
| Student elicits further information about the patient's occupation |
| Student elicits further information about any prescribed medication |
| Student elicits further information about over-the-counter medication |
| Student elicits further information about remedies tried |
| Student elicits further information about past medical history |
| Student elicits further information about family history |

(*continued*)

---

**MARKING CRITERIA – SKIN/ECZEMA ON HANDS**

Student elicits further information about other family members with similar symptoms

Student asks about products used, e.g. gloves

Student asks about contraception, e.g. condoms

Student asks about hobbies

Student asks about pets

Student asks about the patient's history of smoking

Student asks about the patient's use of alcohol

Student asks about the patient's use of recreational drugs

Student establishes any concerns of the patient related to their occupation

Student considers possible differential diagnoses, e.g.
- contact dermatitis/eczema
- infected eczema
- scabies

---

## Paediatric history taking

You may sometimes be asked to undertake a history taking station for a child and their carer, even if you are not undertaking a paediatric-focused course. This is because many nurse practitioner students will be working in an area where contact with children is likely, such as primary healthcare. A paediatric history taking station does not normally use a child as the actual patient, but instead would use someone playing the role of the carer and an age-appropriate child-sized mannequin in place of a child. As this is a role play situation you should attempt to interact with the carer and mannequin as you would do normally in clinical practice in order to demonstrate your genuine ability to interact with both the carer and their child.

Common scenarios that may be used for a paediatric history taking station include a child presenting with a fever, a child presenting with a rash and a child presenting with diarrhoea and vomiting. Unless you are undertaking a paediatric-focused course, most paediatric OSCE scenarios feature a child aged from 2 years old and above.

In contrast to adult history taking, paediatric history taking requires a greater number of comprehensive questions to cover all the potential medical problems a child may present with. Typical examples of problem-focused questions include:
- a history of fever, including duration and response to antipyretics (if used)
- ear, nose and throat symptoms such as a sore throat or earache
- respiratory symptoms such as cough, wheezing or breathlessness

- abdominal symptoms such as urinary problems, abdominal pain, diarrhoea, vomiting and bowel function: in younger children the effect of the presenting problem on their urine output needs to be considered
- assessing possible skin symptoms such as rashes
- food and fluid intake: has this been affected by the presenting problem? In younger children breast-feeding versus bottle feeding must be discerned
- contact with other children who may have had similar symptoms: are other family members/close contacts affected?
- any relevant travel history.

### ⮕ Red flags
- Fever history (if not already covered).
- Potential meningitis symptoms, such as a worsening headache, light sensitivity, neck pain or stiffness, associated vomiting, and a non-blanching rash.
- Whether the carer has noted a rapid deterioration in the child's condition, such as a decreased response or floppiness.

Examples of background questions to explore include:
- any past history of previous similar problems
- past medical history including birth and neonatal history
- drug history (including usage of over-the-counter and alternative medicines)
- completion of vaccinations schedule
- allergies
- dietary pattern
- social history, including status of attending carer (e.g. parent or legal guardian), family structure, childcare usage (e.g. a childminder or a nursery); in older children school attendance should be also be considered
- potential exposure to tobacco smoke at home (particularly relevant for ear, nose, throat and respiratory problems)
- the carer's ideas and concerns about the child's presenting problem and their expectations for treatment.

**TABLE 4.12** Marking criteria for paediatric history taking OSCE – 3-year-old child with a rash

| MARKING CRITERIA PAEDIATRIC HISTORY TAKING |
| --- |

Student introduces self to patient

Student uses open-ended questions appropriately

Student elicits why the patient has attended

Student allows the carer to explain the signs and symptoms without interruption

**Presenting symptoms**

Student explores rash symptom

Student asks how and where it started

Student asks what it looked like at the start

Student asks what it looks like now

Student asks if it is itchy

Student asks if there are any associated symptoms, specifically

- fever
- red eyes
- upper respiratory tract infection
- joint pains

Student explores unwell symptoms

Student elicits when the problem started

Student elicits if anyone else close to the patient has been ill with a similar problem

Student elicits other provoking factors, e.g. drugs, allergens, pets, insects, heat

Student elicits relieving factors, e.g. paracetamol, antihistamine, topical treatments

Student establishes the effect of the symptoms on activities of daily living (eating, drinking, playing, sleeping)

Student asks if there are any other associated problems

Student asks about the patient's general activity level

Student asks about the patient's eating and drinking

Student asks about the patient's urine output

**►❶► Red flags**

Student asks if the rash is non-blanching

Student asks if the child is immuno-compromised

Student asks if the child is ill, toxic or febrile

Student asks if there has been a rapid decline in the child's condition

Student asks about contacts with pregnant women

**Past medical history/family history**

Student establishes the child's past medical history (including immunisation history)

Student asks about the child's family history

*(continued)*

---

MARKING CRITERIA PAEDIATRIC HISTORY TAKING

---

**Lifestyle/social history**

Student asks about the child's home circumstances

Student asks about the child's family members

Student asks about the child's day care arrangements

Student asks about the child's diet

**Medication/allergies**

Student asks about the child's medications including prescribed, over-the-counter, and alternative

Student asks about the child's allergies

**Self-help**

Student elicits any self-help to date

**Ideas, concerns and expectations**

Student establishes what the carer thinks is wrong

---

## History taking OSCE stations in summary

The key to success in OSCE history taking is practising, whether you do this in your clinical setting, with student colleagues, or with friends and family. Adjoined to this emphasis on practising is the need to ensure that you commit to memory a structured sequence for problem-focused history taking, such as the one detailed below:

### Generic summary sequence for problem-focused history taking in an OSCE

- Introduce yourself.
- Ask the patient/carer how you can help them.
- Find out what the patient's presenting complaint is.

### Take a focused history of the presenting complaint

- The OPQRSTU mnemonic can give you a structured format
  — **O**ther symptoms/**O**thers affected
  — **P**rovocative/**P**alliative
  — **Q**uality/**Q**uantity
  — **R**egion/**R**adiation
  — **S**everity/**S**ymptoms
  — **T**iming/**T**reatment
  — What do **U** think the problem is?/What do **U** want to do about it?

➤❗➤   **Red flags** related to the patient's presenting complaint
- Similar problems in past/related medical history.

**Background questions including:**
- past medical history
- drug history
- allergies
- family history
- social history
- exercise
- smoking
- alcohol
- recreational drugs
- new sexual contacts/regular partner/previous screening
- menstrual history/risk of pregnancy (this would be a **red flag** in abdominal pain history taking).

## References

1 Douglas G, Nicol F, Robertson C, editors. *Macleod's Clinical Examination*. 11th ed. Edinburgh: Churchill Livingstone; 2005.
2 Thomas J, Monaghan T, editors. *Oxford Handbook of Clinical Examination and Practical Skills*. Oxford: Oxford University Press; 2007.

## Further reading

Bickley L, Szilagyi P. *Bates' Guide to Physical Examination and History Taking*. 9th ed. London: Lippincott; 2007.
Hastings A. The consultation. In: Hastings A, Redsell S, editors. *The Good Consultation Guide for Nurses*. Oxford: Radcliffe Publishing; 2006. pp. 15–29.
Hopcroft K, Forte V. *Symptom Sorter*. 3rd ed. Oxford: Radcliffe Publishing; 2007.

# 5

# Physical examination OSCE stations

## The purpose of physical examination OSCE stations

Physical examination stations are designed to objectively assess your ability to undertake a structured physical examination of a patient presenting with one or more common medical complaints. Physical examination OSCEs may sometimes be linked to an OSCE history taking scenario or alternatively they may be designed as discrete stations. In a physical examination station which is not linked to a history taking station you will normally be given a brief history scenario complaint, which should help you establish the selected physical examination you will need to complete. An example of a brief history scenario would be: 'This 38-year-old patient has come to see you today because they have had a productive cough, with green coloured phlegm for 4 days'. This scenario should prompt you to conduct a respiratory tract examination. You may wish to clarify or verify the patient's brief history, but you should not do this at the expense of conducting the requisite physical examination. While focused history taking helps to identify possible differential diagnoses for a patient's presenting problem, structured physical examination of a patient is used to help either refute or support a tentative differential diagnosis. As with history taking stations it is possible that at the end of your examination you may be asked to give a list of possible differential diagnoses relevant to the OSCE scenario.

## Key activities to undertake in a physical examination station

In a physical examination station you need to be able to demonstrate competence in using advanced practice physical examination skills such as inspection, palpation, percussion and auscultation. These skills need to be applied as indicated by the patient's presenting problem. You would not normally be asked to examine a patient from head to toe, unless you are taking part in a top-to-toe physical examination, which usually occurs at the end of intensive short courses covering physical examination skills training. Remember that sometimes in the haste to demonstrate new advanced practice skills you can sometimes forget other essential activities, such as saying that you would record and interpret the patient's vital signs (you would not normally be expected to actually record the vital signs, as pre-determined competence in this area is implicit in your registration as a nurse). A selective application of the physical examination skills of inspection, palpation, percussion and auscultation is required in relation to the parts of the OSCE patient's body system requiring examination. A brief review of each of these activities is presented below.

**Inspection**

This is the most frequently used technique of physical examination. It begins as soon as you meet your patient, before they realise that you have your clinical gaze upon them, so as to ensure a full range of observation which should continue throughout the duration of the OSCE station. Inspection is divided into general and specific inspection. General inspection gives you an overview impression of the patient's physical and psychological status, and should include observation of the patient's demeanour, their clothing and general appearance, skin colour/skin condition, and any signs of immediate distress such as breathlessness, discomfort, sweating or pallor. General inspection may also include, as needed, inspection of the patient's hands, eyes, lips and mouth. Potential locomotor problems such as back pain will also require inspection of the patient's gait.

A specific inspection of a patient's problem area, for example their chest if they are presenting with a cough, provides additional information about the patient. A specific inspection often requires the removal of some parts of the patient's clothing. For example, patients must remove their top clothes (in women leaving their bra in place) during the OSCE station if you need to inspect a patient's chest. Once the problem area has been uncovered you should observe it for symmetry, unusual swellings/lumps, redness, skin lesions, scars, rashes and, if there is a trauma-related history, signs of injury. If the patient is experiencing pain you can also ask them to indicate their perceived area of discomfort. Comparative observations should also be made of the affected versus the unaffected area of the body; such as comparing knees in a patient presenting with a painful knee.

Both general and specific inspection requires good ambient lighting which should already be in place during your OSCE station. However a specific inspection may sometimes also require the use of additional directional lighting, such as a pen torch or an otoscope light. This equipment should be provided at a physical examination OSCE station, but you need to decide when to use it. Common examples of using directional lighting include assessing pupil reactions or measuring the jugular venous pressure. Specific inspection may also sometimes require the use of diagnostic instruments to enhance your view of the patient's body, such as an ophthalmoscope or a speculum. Again, these items of equipment should be provided at your OSCE station.

## Palpation

Palpation requires you to therapeutically touch the patient with your hands, using different degrees of pressure. Palpation ideally requires short fingernails and warm, dry hands (though this may be difficult to achieve if you are nervous or if the OSCE takes place on a cold day). Palpation can be used to investigate further any abnormalities, such as pain, swellings or skin lesions that you have noted on inspection or identified in the history. Palpation may be divided into light palpation and deep palpation. Light palpation is typically used to identify an area of swelling or tenderness, or to mark out the parameters of a lesion, or to assess neurovascular status, such as sensations or capillary refill. Deep palpation is used after light palpation to identify masses or to further assess degrees of tenderness. Comparative palpation of the patient's unaffected side may sometimes be required to assess their normal palpable surface anatomy. The right amount of pressure must applied to the patient when palpating an area; if it is too light you will not be able to illicit any findings, if it is too deep you will cause discomfort to the patient.

## Percussion

Percussion involves tapping the patient's skin with your fingers or hands to assess underlying anatomical structures and related pathological findings. Percussion is commonly used in chest and abdominal examinations to detect the presence of air, fluid or solids. This assessment is achieved through eliciting different percussion notes such as resonance, tympany and dullness. Through percussion you can approximately discern the location, size and density of the underlying structure you are examining. Percussion is a skill that many students find difficult to achieve both for eliciting an audible effective percussion note, and also for interpreting an elicited percussion note. You should therefore practise percussion before an OSCE so that you can effectively elicit an audible percussion note when examining your OSCE patient, and also so that you can correctly discriminate and interpret the percussion notes you elicit in relation to the patient's presenting problem.

### Auscultation
Auscultation involves listening to sounds produced by the body, such as heart sounds, blood vessels, breath sounds and bowel sounds. These sounds may be heard directly by the unaided ear, (such as in a patient with asthma presenting with an audible wheeze) or indirectly through an acoustic stethoscope. Auscultation requires practise to be able to distinguish normal and abnormal body sounds. In addition, practise using a quality stethoscope is recommended, as this will augment your auscultatory ability during the OSCE. A quality stethoscope is normally be provided for you at the OSCE station or alterna--tively, if you prefer, it is possible to use your own stethoscope. Auscultation is mostly used in medical diagnosis during a chest examination (breath sounds), an abdominal examination (bowel sounds) and a cardiac examination (heart and arterial sounds). In addition to auscultating the problem area of your OSCE patient you may sometimes be required to listen to audio recordings of auscultatory sounds either via speakers, electronic stethoscopes or in clinical simulation mannequins. These audio recordings are normally linked to the OSCE patient's presenting problem and you would be expected to correctly identify their contextual clinical meaning.

## Examples of specific physical examination sequences to learn in relation to different body systems
These examples should be interpreted flexibly in conjunction with the recommended physical examination textbook cited by your university.

## Ear, nose and throat physical examination
A typical physical examination OSCE scenario would be a patient presenting with a sore throat or an earache.
General inspection
- Are there any immediate signs of distress?
- Is there any drooling of saliva?
- Is there audible respiratory stridor?
- Is there asymmetry of head or neck features?

Vital signs
- At the minimum, check the temperature and pulse.
- In a child also check the respiratory rate.

Mouth
- Inspect lips for colour and moisture, swelling, lumps, cracks, vesicles, crusts.
- Inspect gums and teeth. Note any gum swelling, redness, dental decay, loose teeth, missing teeth, dental prostheses.
- Inspect oral mucosa and tongue, noting any unusual markings, ulcers, white patches or plaques, lumps or nodules.
- Inspect the hard palate (common site of Kaposi's sarcoma).
- Inspect salivary ducts: Stenson's (parotid ducts) and Wharton's (submaxillary ducts).

Throat
- Ask the patient to say 'Ah' and note soft palate rising on phonation – may need to use tongue depressor (phonation is controlled by cranial nerve X [CNX]).
- Inspect soft palate, pillars, uvula, tonsils and pharynx, noting any exudate, tonsil enlargement, uvula midline deviation, ulcers, drooling, or halitosis.

Nose (external)
- Inspect the external nose for symmetry, redness, swelling, lumps, and lesions such as vesicles or yellow crusting.
- Palpate the nasal bone and tip for tenderness.

Nostrils
- Apply gentle pressure on tip of nose and push upwards. This opens up nostrils.
- Inspect nasal vestibules with light.
- For an internal exam use an auroscope and a large speculum – inspect mucosa, turbinates and septum.

Sinuses
- Inspect the face for sinus area swelling.
- Palpate frontal and maxillary sinuses in turn, checking for tenderness.
- Ask the patient to lean forward to see if a sinus pressure sensation is elicited.

Ears (external)
- Inspect outer ears for swelling, redness, lumps, discharge, and skin lesions.
- Palpate tragus (often tender in otitis externa).

- Perform ear tug (causes pain in otitis externa).
- Palpate mastoid process, looking for tenderness.
- Tenderness behind the ear often occurs in otitis media.

Ears (otoscope)
- Turn on the bright light on the otoscope. Start with the unaffected ear for comparison.
- Pull ear upwards and backwards in adults or downwards in children.
- Use largest possible ear speculum.
- Insert gently in external auditory méatus.
- Inspect the canal looking for pain on insertion, redness, swelling, discharge, foreign bodies and wax.
- Inspect the tympanic membrane for its normal anatomical landmarks: cone of light, umbo, handle of malleus, pars flaccida, pars tensa, and annulus.
- Inspect the tympanic membrane for abnormalities, such as redness, fluid, bulging, perforation, scarring, retraction, opacity, or the presence of grommets.

Neck glands
Systematically palpate the head and neck lymph nodes looking for signs of lymphadenopathy (swelling and/or tenderness)
- occipital – base of skull
- posterior auricular – behind the ear
- preauricular – in front of ear
- tonsillar – at angle of mandible
- submandibular – midway between angle and tip of mandible
- submental – midline tip of mandible
- superficial cervical – superficial to sternocleidomastoid
- posterior cervical – along posterior edge of sternocleidomastoid
- deep cervical – deep in sternocleidomastoid.

---

**Summary sequence for ear, nose and throat examination**
- Perform a general inspection
- Examine vital signs
- Inspect external ears
- Palpate external ears
- Perform auroscope examination
- Inspect external nose

---

○ Palpate nose
○ Perform light examination (otoscope) of nostrils
○ Inspect and palpate maxillary and frontal sinuses
○ Inspect outer lips
○ Inspect gums and teeth
○ Inspect mouth and salivary ducts
○ Inspect soft palate, pillars, uvula, tonsils, and pharynx
○ Inspect CNX – observe soft palate rise on phonation
○ Palpate head and neck lymph nodes.

**TABLE 5.1** OSCE marking criteria for an adult ear, nose and throat examination

| MARKING CRITERIA – EAR, NOSE AND THROAT |
| --- |
| Student's general approach to patient: introduces self, shows warmth, keeps eye contact, provides patient with adequate explanation |
| Student says they will take the patient's temperature |
| Student performs general inspection of patient, including any signs of distress |
| Student inspects external ears bilaterally |
| Student palpates external pinna and tragus bilaterally to elicit pain, or to identify masses |
| Student palpates mastoid bones bilaterally |
| Student observes ear canal and tympanic membrane bilaterally using a safe otoscope technique |
| Student names landmarks, i.e., light reflex, umbo, malleus, pars tensa |
| Student inspects both nostrils and lower/middle turbinates |
| Student palpates frontal sinuses |
| Student palpates maxillary sinuses |
| Student inspects mouth and pharynx |
| Student looks for redness, swelling and exudate in throat |
| Student observes tonsils and uvula |
| Student palpates relevant lymph nodes for swelling and tenderness<br>• preauricular<br>• posteria auricular<br>• superficial cervical<br>• posterior cervical<br>• deep cervical<br>• tonsillar<br>• submandibular<br>• submental |

## Respiratory chest physical examination

A typical scenario for this type of station would be to assess a patient presenting with a cough.

General inspection

- How does the patient appear?
- Does the patient show any immediate signs of distress?
- Assess perfusion.
- Listen to any audible breathing sounds.
- Inspect the neck for accessory muscle usage and signs of tracheal deviation.
- Assess speech; is the patient able to speak in full sentences?
- Assess fingers for signs of clubbing, cyanosis or nicotine staining.

Vital signs

- At the minimum, inspect the patient's respiratory rate, pulse, temperature and, if available, oxygen saturation.
- Also inspect the peak expiratory flow rate in patients with asthma or wheezing.

Preparation of patient for the examination

- Patient should be undressed (top only).
- Examine the patient in a good light.
- Remember to compare the patient's chest walls (anterior > posterior > lateral).
- Think about the surface anatomy of the thorax.
- Start with posterior chest (patient sitting up) and move to anterior chest (patient either supine or sitting up).

Chest inspection

- Note the shape of the chest.
- Check for deformities or asymmetry.
- Note any skin marks, scars or lesions.
- Note the respiratory pattern – rate, rhythm, depth and effort.
- Observe the patient's use of accessory muscles/interspaces retraction.
- Note any impaired respiratory movements in the patient.

Palpation

- Palpate the patient's ribs and intercostal spaces.
- Palpate each chest side in turn – remember the lateral chest walls.
- Identify any areas of palpable tenderness.

Chest expansion (one side of chest only required)
- Place thumbs at costal margin (anterior) or 10th rib level (posterior).
- Fingers on lateral rib cage.
- Slide hands medially to raise a skin fold between your thumbs.
- Ask the patient to inhale deeply.
- Note divergence and symmetry of thumb movement as chest expands.

Tactile fremitus
- Assesses palpable vibrations transmitted through the bronchopulmonary tree to the chest wall as the patient speaks.
- Place the ball or ulnar surface of hand on the patient's chest wall as the patient says '99'.
- Your hand placement should be two places anterior: one place laterally (anterior chest), and three places posterior: one place laterally (posterior chest).
- Identify any areas of increased, decreased or absent fremitus.
- Fremitus normally decreases as you move down the chest wall.

Percussion
- This is an important feature of the chest exam.
- It is a technique to establish whether the underlying tissues are air-filled, fluid-filled or solid.
- This technique requires practice.
- Percuss the intercostal spaces on one side of the chest and then the other at the same level.
- Percuss in four symmetrical places anterior and two laterally, and five symmetrical places posterior and two laterally.
- The normal dominant percussion note is resonance. Dullness occurs over organs (heart/liver) and areas of consolidation or masses.

Auscultation
- This is technique for assessing the air flow through the chest.
- It involves listening to the sounds generated by breathing and also listening for any added (adventitious) breath sounds.
- Use the diaphragm of the stethoscope in auscultation.
- Ask the patient to breath deeply through their open mouth.
- Auscultate over the intercostal spaces on one side of the chest and then the other at same level. Start at the apices of the chest.
- Auscultate in four symmetrical places anterior and two laterally, and five symmetrical places posterior and two laterally.

- Compare the sounds from side to side.
- Listen to at least one full breath cycle in each location.
- Be aware of the patient potentially hyperventilating.
- The dominant normal breath sounds are vesicular breath sounds, where inspiration sounds longer than expiration; these are heard over most of the lung fields.
- Other breath sounds are bronchovesicular, where the inspiration equals the expiration. These are normally heard over the first and second intercostal spaces and between the scapulae.
- Bronchial breath sounds are when the expiration sounds are longer than inspiration. These are normally heard over the manubrium.

Added (adventitious breath sounds)
- Displaced bronchovesicular/bronchial breath sounds (consolidation).
- Crackles – fine or coarse (pneumonia, lower respiratory tract infection).
- Wheezes – high pitched (asthma, chronic obstructive pulmonary disease, infection).
- Rhonchi – low pitched (secretions, infection).
- Pleural rub – grating in one area (pleural effusion).

---

### Summary sequence for respiratory chest examination

- General inspection of patient
- Vital signs (respiratory rate, temperature, pulse)
- Chest inspection
- Chest expansion (anterior or posterior)
- Palpate chest
- Tactile fremitus
- Percussion
- Auscultation.

---

**TABLE 5.2** OSCE marking criteria for an adult chest respiratory examination

| MARKING CRITERIA – RESPIRATORY CHEST |
| --- |
| Student's general approach to patient: introduces self, shows warmth, keeps eye contact, provides patient with adequate explanation |
| Student says they will take the temperature, pulse and respiratory rate |
| Student performs general inspection of patient; including perfusion, and signs of respiratory distress |

*(continued)*

---

**MARKING CRITERIA – RESPIRATORY CHEST**

---

Student checks fingers for signs of smoking, clubbing and cyanosis

Student inspects the chest fully exposed, observing: chest symmetry and shape, trachea in midline, respiratory movements (equal right and left, *respiratory rate* and rhythm)

Student measures chest expansion, using hands on *either* the anterior *or* posterior chest

Student palpates
- for fremitus, comparing sides

Student percusses
- anterior chest, comparing sides
- posterior chest, comparing sides

Student auscultates
- anterior chest, comparing sides
- posterior chest, comparing sides

---

## Cardiac and peripheral vascular examination

Common OSCE scenarios are the assessment of a patient presenting with breathlessness, chest pain or palpitations.

General inspection
- How does the patient appear?
- Does the patient show any immediate signs of distress, for example, pallor, shortness of breath, sweating?
- Assess perfusion.
- Assess fingers for signs of clubbing, cyanosis or nicotine staining.
- Face – check for xanthelasma.
- Eyes – check for corneal arcus.
- Mouth – check for signs of dental decay, ulcers or other mouth lesions.

Vital signs
- At the minimum check blood pressure, respiratory rate, pulse, temperature and, if available, oxygen saturation.

Peripheral vascular system (skin)
- Inspect and palpate upper limbs, hands and nails: temperature, moisture, colour, oedema, venous pattern, absence of lesions, capillary refill, clubbing, splinter haemorrhages.
- Inspect and palpate lower limbs, feet and nails: as above, also varicosities, pigmentation and hair distribution.
- Check for peripheral oedema.

Peripheral vascular system (pulses)
- radial (brachial)
- femoral
- popliteal
- posterior tibial
- dorsalis pedis
- palpate all pulses, noting and comparing rate, rhythm, amplitude and equality.

Assessing the jugular venous pulse
- Inspect the neck vessels looking at internal jugular vein, which runs between the two heads (sternal and clavicular) of the sternocleidomastoid muscle and up in front of the ear.
- You cannot normally see the internal jugular vein itself, but you can see its pulsation.
- The jugular venous pulse reflects right atrial pressure and is an important measure of cardiac function.
- Approach the patient from the right side.
- Position the person supine at 30 to 45°.
- Turn the person's head slightly away from the examined side, and direct a strong directional light obliquely across the neck.
- Note the external jugular veins overlying the sternomastoid muscle.
- Now look for the pulsation of the internal jugular vein in the triangular area between the sternal and clavicular borders of the sternocleidomastoid muscle above the clavicle.
- The internal jugular pulse is normally located lower, and is more lateral than the higher and medially located carotid pulse.
- It is undulant, with two visible waves, while the carotid is brisk, with one wave.
- It varies with respiration; its level may descend during inspiration.
- The internal jugular pulse is not normally palpable.

Assessing the jugular venous pressure
- To estimate the jugular venous pressure you need to find the highest point of oscillation in the right internal jugular vein.
- The jugular venous pressure is usually measured in centimetres vertical distance above the sternal angle, with the patient placed at an angle between 30 to 45°.
- The normal jugular venous pressure is 2 to 3 cm above the sternal angle.

Assessing the carotid pulse
- Inspect the neck for carotid pulsations.
- Palpate separately each carotid artery medial to the sternocleidomastoid muscle with your thumbs.
- Feel the contour and amplitude of the pulses (you may also feel a thrill).
- Auscultate both carotid arteries for bruits.

Inspection and palpation of the precordium
- Inspect the anterior chest. You may be able to note the apical impulse. Also note the absence of heaves or lifts.
- Locate and palpate the apical impulse, or point of maximal impulse, medial to midclavicular line at 4th or 5th intercostal space.
- If you cannot readily locate the apex beat ask the patient to lie on their left side, exhale and hold their breath.
- Palpate the left sternal border and base for impulses and thrills.

Auscultation of the precordium
Auscultate, with the diaphragm pressed firmly, in the following sequence:
- right 2nd intercostal space (ICS) (aortic) followed by
- left 2nd ICS (pulmonic) followed by
- left 3rd ICS followed by
- left 4th ICS followed by
- left 5th ICS (tricuspid) followed by
- apex 5th ICS at midclavicular line (mitral).

Switch to the bell held lightly at the apex and repeat the previous sequence in reverse:
- apex 5th ICS midclavicular (mitral) followed by
- left 5th ICS (tricuspid) followed by
- left 4th ICS followed by
- left 3rd ICS followed by
- left 2nd ICS (pulmonic) followed by
- right 2nd ICS (aortic).

Auscultation special manoeuvres
- Ask the patient to roll partly onto their left side and listen with bell over the apical impulse (sound 3, sound 4, mitral murmurs).
- Ask the patient to sit up, lean forward, exhale and hold their breath, then listen with the diaphragm at the lower left sternal border and apex (aortic murmur).

Listening to the normal heart sounds
- Note the patient's heart rate and rhythm.
- Identify sound 1 and sound 2, which occur as a pair of sounds (lub-dub), with sound 1 the first of the pair.
- Sound 1 is louder than sound 2 at the apex; sound 2 is louder than sound 1 at the base.
- Sound 1 coincides with the carotid artery pulse.

---

**Summary sequence for peripheral vascular and cardiac examination**

○ Perform general inspection.
○ Inspect vital signs (blood pressure, pulse, respiratory rate).
○ Inspect and palpate upper limbs, hands and nails.
○ Inspect and palpate lower limbs, feet, and nails.
○ Inspect and measure jugular venous pressure.
○ Inspect and auscultate carotid pulses.
○ Inspect the precordium.
○ Locate and palpate the apical impulse.
○ Palpate the precordium for impulses and thrills.
○ Auscultate the precordium with diaphragm: right 2nd intercostal space (ICS), left 2nd ICS, left 3rd ICS, left 4th ICS, left 5th ICS, apex; and then repeat sequence in reverse with bell.
○ Ask the patient to roll onto their left side and then listen with bell over apex (sound 3, sound 4, and mitral murmurs).
○ Ask the patient to sit up, lean forward and exhale, and then listen with diaphragm over lower left sternal border and apex (aortic murmur).

---

**TABLE 5.3** OSCE marking criteria for a cardiovascular examination

| MARKING CRITERIA – CARDIOVASCULAR |
|---|
| Student's general approach to patient: introduces self, shows warmth, keeps eye contact, provides patient with adequate explanation |
| Student explains the procedure to the patient |
| Student observes the patient's face for colour, xanthelasma |
| Student inspects the patient's skin and nails for warmth, colour, sweating, clubbing and splinter haemorrhages |
| Student takes the patient's radial pulse for rate and rhythm, also measures blood pressure and respiratory rate |
| Student says they will take an accurate blood pressure using the correct technique |

*(continued)*

---

MARKING CRITERIA – CARDIOVASCULAR

---

Student makes patient lie at a 45° and exposes the patient's chest

Student assesses jugular venous pressure

Student palpates the carotid artery

Student listens for carotid bruits with the stethoscope

Student inspects for ankle oedema

Student inspects precordium for apical impulse

Student palpates chest wall for apical impulse

Student palpates chest wall for thrills/heaves

Student auscultates in correct areas for heart sounds

Student performs special manoeuvres and specifies where listening
- with patient sitting up right
- with patient lying on left side

---

## Abdominal physical examination

Common OSCE scenarios for abdominal physical examination are acute onset abdominal pain, abdominal pain with urinary symptoms, abdominal pain with vaginal symptoms, or upper abdominal pain symptoms, such as dyspepsia.

General inspection
- Are there any obvious signs of discomfort or distress such as pallor or sweating?
- Assess the peripheries – check fingers for perfusion and clubbing.
- Check the patient's mouth for integrity of oral mucosa and signs of dehydration.

Vital signs
- At a minimum check the patient's blood pressure, pulse and temperature. You may also need to include the patient's respiratory rate, particularly in children.

Preparation for examination
- Ensure that the patient has an empty bladder.
- Ask the patient to lie down on the couch or bed with their arms folded across their chest or relaxed at their sides, and place a pillow (if available) under their head.
- Explain the sequence of the examination.
- Ensure the abdomen is adequately exposed – from the xiphoid process to symphysis pubis.
- Remember to stand at the patient's right side.

Inspection of the abdomen
- Inspect the abdomen from all angles.
- Observe the skin for any scars, striae, rashes or skin lesions.
- Inspect the abdominal contour. Is it flat, rounded, or swollen?
- Observe for abdominal wall symmetry – note any possible areas of asymmetrical enlargement.
- Note any peristaltic waves or aortic pulsations.
- Ask patient to indicate their perceived area of abdominal discomfort.

Percussion
- Percuss lightly in all four abdominal quadrants, noting tympany or dullness. Tympany is the normal dominant percussion note.
- Large areas of dullness may indicate a mass or enlarged organ.
- If this is indicated by the patient's presenting problem, measure the liver span at right midclavicular line costal margin using percussion. The normal liver span ranges from 6 to 12 cm.

Light palpation
- Use fingers together and flat on abdominal wall.
- Palpate aorta, noting pulsation and width.
- Lightly palpate in all four quadrants to identify areas of tenderness and muscular guarding.
- Note any palpable organs or masses.
- Observe for abdominal muscle wall guarding.

Deep palpation
- Use deep palpitation to identify abdominal masses and other abnormalities.
- Also use it to further assess previously identified areas of tenderness.
- Use a technique of two-handed deep palpation in all four abdominal quadrants.
- Observe again for abdominal muscle wall guarding.

Rebound tenderness
- Check rebound tenderness to assess for possible inflammation of the peritoneum.
- Check in areas of previously identified pain or tenderness.
- After deep palpation, press your fingers in firmly and slowly and then quickly withdraw them.

- Which hurts the patient more? Pressing or letting go?
- A withdrawal pain equals rebound tenderness.

Liver palpation (if indicated by the patient's presenting problem)
- The liver edge is not always palpable.
- Liver palpation is used to check for tenderness, firmness and rounding or irregularity of the liver edge.
- Place your left hand underneath patient at the right 11/12th rib level.
- Press your right hand on the patient's right abdominal lateral/rectus muscle, below the percussed border of liver dullness.
- Ask the patient to take a deep breath in and out as you palpate the liver edge.

Spleen palpation (if indicated by the patient's presenting problem)
- The spleen tip is not normally palpable.
- With your left hand, reach over and press underneath the patient at the lower left rib cage.
- Place your right hand below the left costal margin and press in towards spleen as the patient takes a deep breath in and out.
- Note splenic tenderness and contour, and estimate the distance between the spleen tip and the costal margin.
- Repeat palpation with the patient lying on their right side with knees flexed.

Kidney palpation (if indicated by the patient's presenting problem)
- The kidney is palpable in some people, such as teenagers and older people with a loss of muscle bulk.
- Left kidney – reach over and press your left hand underneath at costal margin.
- Place your right hand in the left upper quadrant and press down as the patient takes a deep breath and then exhales.
- You may feel the kidney slip back in your hands.
- If the kidney is palpable, note its size, shape, contour and tenderness.
- Right kidney – place your left hand underneath at costal margin.
- Place right hand in right upper quadrant and press down.
- Proceed as for left kidney.

Auscultation of abdomen (students using certain American physical examination textbooks may be more familiar with auscultation being done after abdominal wall inspection)

- Use diaphragm to listen to bowel sounds in all four quadrants.
- If indicated by the patient's presentation, use the bell of the stethoscope to listen for arterial bruits (vascular sounds) over the aorta and renal, iliac and femoral arteries.

Inguinal nodes (you may not be asked to do this in your actual OSCE for reasons of modesty, but you may be asked how you would palpate the nodes and what the normal findings should be)
- Check for enlarged nodes with or without tenderness (lymphadenopathy).
- Check right and left side superficial inguinal nodes, both horizontal and vertical chains.
- The inguinal nodes may not normally be palpable.
- If they are palpable note their size, consistency and tenderness, and whether they are discrete.
- Note the absence of hernias.

Additional technique to assess for kidney tenderness
- Indirect (fist) percussion of left and right costovertebral angles.
- Place the palmar surface of one hand in the costovertebral angle and strike it firmly with the ulnar surface of your fist. Repeat for the other kidney.
- Note any tenderness on indirect percussion that may indicate the inflammation of the renal parenchyma.

---

**Summary sequence for abdominal examination**
- ○ Perform a general inspection of the patient.
- ○ Check vital signs (blood pressure, pulse, temperature).
- ○ Inspect the abdomen.
- ○ Percuss all four quadrants.
- ○ Percuss the liver span.
- ○ Lightly palpate all four quadrants.
- ○ Deeply palpate all four quadrants.
- ○ Check for rebound tenderness in areas of pain.
- ○ Palpate the liver, spleen and kidneys.
- ○ Auscultate for bowel sounds in all four quadrants.
- ○ Auscultate for bruits at aorta, renal, iliac, and (femoral) arteries.
- ○ (Inguinal node palpation).
- ○ Indirectly percuss the kidneys.

---

**TABLE 5.4** OSCE marking criteria for abdominal physical examination in a patient presenting with lower abdominal pain and urinary symptoms

| MARKING CRITERIA – ABDOMINAL EXAMINATION |
| --- |
| Student's general approach to patient: introduces self, shows warmth, keeps eye contact, provides patient with adequate explanation |
| Student says that they will take vital signs |
| Student undertakes a general inspection of the patient |
| Student explains examination sequence to patient |
| Student asks the patient to expose their abdomen from the xiphoid sternum to the suprapubic area for the examination |
| Student inspects the abdomen for shape, symmetry, scars, swellings, skin lesions and abdominal wall movements |
| Student asks the patient to indicate the area of abdominal pain |
| Student auscultates with stethoscope all four quadrants of diaphragm for presence of bowel sounds |
| Student percusses all four quadrants using a technique that elicits audible tympanic or dull percussion notes |
| Student palpates lightly in all four quadrants and starts away from the indicated area of pain |
| Student palpates deeply in all four quadrants and starts away from the indicated area of pain |
| Student observes the patient's face for signs of pain during light and deep palpation |
| Student checks for rebound tenderness |
| Student palpates both kidneys |
| Student indirectly percusses costovertebral angles for kidney tenderness |

## Pelvic examination

A typical OSCE physical examination scenario could be a woman presenting with abdominal pain and unusual vaginal discharge. This station could be linked to abdominal physical examination. Normally a pelvis simulation model is used in place of a patient; however, you should conduct your examination as though you are dealing with a real patient.

General inspection
- Are there any obvious signs of discomfort or distress such as pallor or sweating?

Vital signs
- The minimum check required is the pulse and temperature. Blood pressure and respiratory rate may also be required, depending on the type of presentation.

Preparation of patient
- Explain the purpose and sequence of the examination to the patient and obtain their consent.
- Clearly offer the patient a chaperone to be present during the examination.
- Say that you would check that the patient has passed urine immediately before the examination.
- Say that you would ask the patient to lie down on the couch with her heels together and knees separated with a cover placed over her abdomen.
- Ensure you wear gloves throughout the examination.

External examination
Inspect the:
 — pubic hair distribution
 — inguinal folds
 — labia majora
 — clitoris.
- Separate the labia majora and inspect the labia minora, urethral meatus and vaginal introitus.
- Note any visible inguinal nodes and any vulval swellings, lumps, papules, pustules, vesicles, ulcers, discharge, skin redness or other lesions.
- Palpate any swellings, lumps or skin lesions to estimate their size and tenderness.
- With the labia separated, ask the patient to strain down and note any bulging of the vaginal introitus, which may indicate a prolapse.

Internal examination
- Use a lubricated speculum, which should be gently inserted into the vagina, at an angle, with the handles pointing towards the woman's right leg.
- Once the speculum has been correctly inserted, rotate it to a horizontal position with the handles pointing downwards towards the couch.
- Gently open the speculum blades and lock them in place with the wheel nut. A directional light will be required for the internal inspection.
- Inspect the vaginal walls and cervix, noting any redness, lesions such as ulcers, bleeding, discharge or foreign bodies.
- If indicated by the patient's presenting problem, say that you would take a high vaginal swab to check for infection.
- To withdraw the speculum, release the wheel nut and hold the blade position while gently pulling it out, observing the vaginal mucosa as you

do so. Close the blades as the speculum is withdrawn from the vaginal introitus.

Bimanual examination

- Gently insert your lubricated right index and middle fingers into the vagina. Note any irregularities of the vaginal surface.
- Palpate the cervix in the upper part of vagina noting any tenderness (cervical excitation) that may indicate infection.
- Now place your fingers behind the cervix and with your left hand push down on the pelvic area to note the uterine size, contour, shape and signs of tenderness.
- Finally, palpate the lateral space (fornix) on each side of the cervix while pushing down with your left hand to note any enlargement or tenderness of the ovaries or fallopian tubes.

---

### Summary sequence for pelvic physical examination

○ Perform a general inspection.
○ Check vital signs (blood pressure, pulse, temperature).
○ Explain the examination and obtain the patient's consent to proceed.
○ Offer the patient a chaperone.
○ Inspect the external genitalia.
○ Palpate any observed lumps, swellings or lesions.
○ Perform a speculum examination.
○ If required, take a high vaginal swab.
○ Directly palpate the cervix.
○ Perform a bimanual palpation of the uterus, fallopian tubes and ovaries.

---

**TABLE 5.5** OSCE marking criteria for pelvic physical examination in a patient presenting with unusual vaginal discharge

| MARKING CRITERIA – PELVIC EXAMINATION |
| --- |
| Student's general approach to patient: introduces self, shows warmth, keeps eye contact, provides patient with adequate explanation |
| Student explains purpose and sequence of examination to gain patient's consent |
| Student offers the patient a chaperone |
| Student says they would take vital signs |
| Student undertakes a general inspection of the patient |

*(continued)*

MARKING CRITERIA – PELVIC EXAMINATION

Student says that they would ask the patient to expose their pelvic area and cover their abdomen with a drape

Student inspects the external genitalia and groin, noting any visible inguinal nodes, and any vulval swellings, lumps, papules, pustules, vesicles, ulcers, discharge, skin redness or other lesions:
- pubic hair distribution
- inguinal folds
- labia majora
- clitoris
- labia minora
- urethral meatus
- vaginal introitus

Student says they would palpate any observed lumps, swellings or lesions

Student correctly inserts a lubricated speculum for internal examination

Student inspects vaginal walls and cervix using a directional light, noting any redness or lesions such as ulcers, bleeding, discharge, or foreign bodies

Student takes a high vaginal swab as indicated by the patient's presentation

Student correctly removes speculum

Student correctly inserts lubricated index and middle fingers into the vagina for bimanual examination

Student palpates the cervix for tenderness

Student bimanually palpates the uterus

Student bimanually palpates the fallopian tubes and ovaries

## Back and neck musculoskeletal examination

A typical OSCE scenario for this type of station would be a patient presenting with low back pain as a result of indirect trauma, such as heavy lifting.

Remember the musculoskeletal examination sequence of:
- inspection
- palpation
- movement
- selected special tests.

General inspection
- Begin the inspection when you first meet and observe the client and continue doing so during the consultation.
- Remember also to observe the patient discreetly.
- Observe the patient in anterior, posterior and lateral views.
- Check gait – is the patient able to weight bear? Is their gait smooth?
- Exposure of affected area.

Neck inspection
- Ensure the patient's neck and upper back are adequately exposed.
- The patient's head should be erect and the neck held straight.
- Inspect the neck from all aspects (anterior, posterior and lateral).
- Note any obvious swellings or surgical scars.
- Ask the patient to indicate their perceived area of pain.

Neck palpation
- Palpate individual spinous processes of cervical spine to C7/T1 junction.
- Palpate paravertebral muscles on both sides of cervical spine, and also trapezius, and sternocleidomastoid muscles.
- Note any areas of swelling or tenderness.

Neck movements
Observe active range of movement of cervical spine:
- flexion (bending forward)
- extension (bending backwards)
- lateral bending (bending to each side)
- rotation (looking over each shoulder).

Neck resistance movements
Check CN XI (spinal accessory):
- ask the patient to turn their face against your resisting hand (sternomastoid)
- ask the patient to shrug their shoulders against resistance (trapezius).

Neck neurology
- Check upper limbs strengths.
- Check arm reflexes – triceps, biceps, and supinator.
- Check distal sensations.

Back inspection
- Ensure the patient is adequately exposed; their top clothing should be removed, their trousers/skirt loosened, and their sock/tights removed.
- Look for rashes, lesions, curvature, deformity, asymmetry and atrophy.
- Observe the patient bending forward – normal spinal curvature forms a nominal 'c'-shape.
- Check symmetrical height of iliac and sacroiliac crests.
- Ask the patient to indicate their perceived area of pain.

Back palpation
- Palpate spinous processes from T1 to S2.
- Palpate paravertebral muscles on each side of the vertebral column.
- Note areas and levels of tenderness.
- If indicated by the patient's presenting problem check for kidney tenderness by indirect (fist) percussion.

Back movements
Observe the active range of movement of the patient's back.(You may need to stabilise the patient's pelvis by grasping their hips):
- flexion (bending forward)
- extension (bending backwards)
- lateral bending (bending to each side)
- rotation (looking over each shoulder).

Special test – straight leg raise
- This is a test for nerve root irritation caused by a herniated vertebral disc.
- It is especially important to check in patients presenting with low back pain accompanied by pain radiating down the leg.
- Ask the patient to lie supine.
- You should passively raise the patient's straight leg up in the air to the point at which the low back pain occurs.
- If no pain occurs, with the leg still raised, passively dorsiflex the foot.
- If pain occurs, slightly lower the leg until the pain goes and then passively dorsiflex the foot.
- Repeat and compare sides.
- It is normal for slight lower back pain and stretching of hamstrings to occur.
- A positive straight leg raising test occurs with the reproduction of a sharp back pain extending down the leg.
- Passive dorsiflexion of the foot reinforces the pain.

Back neurology
- Check lower limb muscle strengths.
- Check reflexes – knee, ankle and plantar flexion response.
- Check distal sensations.

**Summary sequence for neck and back musculoskeletal examination**

○ Perform general inspection.

○ Observe the patient's gait.

○ Inspect the patient's neck.

○ Palpate the patient's neck.

○ Check the neck movements: extension, flexion, lateral flexion, rotation.

○ Check upper limb muscle strengths, reflexes and distal sensations.

○ Inspect the patient's back.

○ Palpate the patient's back.

○ Check back movements: extension, flexion, lateral flexion, rotation.

○ Straight leg raising (both legs).

○ Check lower limb muscle strengths, reflexes and distal sensations.

**TABLE 5.6** OSCE marking criteria for physical examination of the neck and back in a patient presenting with low back pain

| MARKING CRITERIA – NECK AND BACK PHYSICAL EXAMINATION |
| --- |
| Student shows warm approach to patient |
| Student explains examination procedure to patient |
| Student asks patient to undress to their underwear or shorts to expose their back |
| Student inspects the patient's gait and asks them to walk across room |
| Student inspects the patient's spinal profile and notes curves and symmetry when upright |
| Student inspects the patient's spinal profile when bending forward |
| Student inspects the patient's neck, noting any abnormalities |
| Student palpates the cervical processes of the neck for tenderness |
| Student palpates the patient's neck muscles for tenderness |
| Student performs range of movement on patient's neck<br>• flexion (chin onto chest)<br>• extension (look at the ceiling)<br>• lateral bending (ear to shoulder)<br>• rotation (turn neck through 90° to the right and left) |
| Student palpates spinal processes for tenderness and warmth |
| Student palpates paravertebral muscles for tenderness and warmth |
| Student performs range of movement for back<br>• flexion (bend forwards)<br>• extension (bend backwards)<br>• rotation (turn to the right, then to the left, both with hips stabilised)<br>• lateral bending (to the right and left) |

*(continued)*

---

**MARKING CRITERIA – NECK AND BACK PHYSICAL EXAMINATION**

Student checks straight leg raise in both legs, including ankle dorsiflexion

Student checks lower limb muscle strengths in

- both patient's legs and/or
- checks power in both ankles of
  - plantar flexion
  - dorsiflexion

Student checks lower limb reflexes in both legs (or describes the expected response if a reflex cannot be obtained)

- patella
- ankle
- plantar

---

## Shoulder musculoskeletal examination

An example of a common OSCE scenario for shoulder musculoskeletal examination is a patient presenting with shoulder tip/subacromial pain either after an injury or else occurring after repetitive shoulder movements.

Remember the musculoskeletal examination sequence of:

○ inspection
○ palpation
○ movement
○ selected special tests.

Before you undertake your OSCE review the anatomy of the shoulder, particularly the rotator cuff muscles:

○ **s**upraspinatus
○ **i**nfraspinatus
○ **t**eres minor
○ **s**ubscapularis

  ▷ The rotator cuff acts as a stabiliser for shallow articulation of the humeral head in the glenoid cavity.
  ▷ The subacromial space at the shoulder tip is small and contains the sub-deltoid bursa, and supraspinatus muscle and tendon; hence it is a common site of shoulder pain.

General inspection
Observe for any signs of immediate concern/distress such as:

- suspicion of shoulder dislocation or fracture
- an inability to move the affected shoulder
- evident severe pain
- a distal neurovascular deficit

- Remember other acute causes for shoulder pain such as ischemia or abdominal/pelvic pathologies.

Shoulder inspection
- Expose the upper chest.
- Inspect the patient's neck.
- Compare both shoulders.
- Ask the patient to point to their perceived area of shoulder pain.
- Observe for shoulder shape, symmetry, swelling, deformity, angulation, redness, muscle wasting, scars or skin lesions.

Shoulder palpation:
- suprasternal notch
- sternoclavicular joint, clavicle
- tuberosity of humerus
- coracoid process
- bicipital groove
- scapula
- *rotator cuff muscles:* supraspinatus, infraspinatus, teres minor, subscapularis
- sternomastoid (neck)
- trapezius (neck)
- pectoralis major (upper anterior chest)
- biceps (upper arm)
- deltoid (upper arm)
- triceps (upper arm)
- coracobrachialis (lateral chest)
- lattissimus dorsi (mid-posterior chest).

Arm palpation (sensations)
- Check and compare distal neurovascular status with the unaffected side.
- Check axillary nerve (badge sign).
- Check ulnar nerve.
- Check radial nerve.
- Check median nerve.

Shoulder movements
- Check neck movements first, as detailed above in neck examination.
- Check shoulder flexion (arm forwards).
- Check shoulder extension (arm backwards).
- Check shoulder abduction (arm away from midline).

- Check shoulder adduction (arm towards midline).
- Check lateral (external) rotation (elbow flexed to 90°, tucked into lateral chest wall, and forearm moved away from midline).
- Check medial (internal) rotation (elbow flexed to 90°, tucked into lateral chest wall, and forearm moved towards the midline).

### Selected special tests – shoulder

A large range of special tests for the shoulder are available, many of which are used solely by shoulder specialists. Presented below is a selected range of shoulder tests that are simple to perform and that test all the major problem areas commonly found in the shoulder (rotator cuff muscles, subacromial space, and instability).

Special test 1 – anterior and posterior instability
- Stabilise shoulder from behind and move glenohumeral joint backwards and forwards to assess anterior or posterior instability.
- Compare with unaffected side.
- You are looking for joint laxity in comparison with unaffected side, which can indicate **anterior** or **posterior instability**.

Special test 2 – inferior instability (sulcus sign)
- Stabilise the patient's shoulder from the front and then pull down on the patient's arm to assess inferior instability.
- Compare with unaffected side.
- You are looking for a dip (sulcus) appearing below the acromion, which would indicate **inferior instability**.

Special test 3 – active abduction (painful arc)
- Ask patient to abduct their shoulder.
- Pain occurring between 70–140° may indicate a **subacromial space** problem.
- Pain occurring between 140–80° may indicate an **acromioclavicular joint** problem.

Special test 4 – passive abduction
- Passively abduct the patient's shoulder.
- You are looking for pain occurring around the acromion, which may indicate **subacromial bursitis**.

Special test 5 – resisted abduction
- Ask the patient to abduct their arm while you apply an opposing force.

- Compare their shoulder muscle strength with unaffected side.
- Pain occurring in the superior aspect of the shoulder may indicate **supraspinatus tendonitis**.
- Weakness on resistance may indicate a possible rotator cuff tear (**supraspinatus**).

Special test 6 – resisted lateral rotation
- Ask patient to flex their elbow and press their upper arm into their lateral chest wall, and to move their forearm laterally.
- You should apply an opposing medial force.
- Pain in the posterior aspect of the shoulder may indicate **infraspinatus** or **teres minor tendonitis**.
- Weakness on resistance may indicate a possible rotator cuff tear (**infraspinatus** or **teres minor**).

Special test 7 – resisted medial rotation
- Ask patient to flex their elbow and press their upper arm into their lateral chest wall, and to move their forearm medially.
- You should apply an opposing lateral force.
- Compare with the unaffected side.
- Pain in the anterior aspect of the shoulder may indicate **subscapularis tendonitis**.
- Weakness on resistance may indicate a possible rotator cuff tear (**subscapularis**).

---

**Summary sequence for shoulder musculoskeletal examination**
- Perform general inspection.
- Perform inspection.
- Perform palpation.
- Check shoulder movements: flexion, extension, abduction, adduction, lateral rotation, medial rotation.
- Check anterior and posterior instability.
- Check inferior instability (sulcus sign).
- Check active abduction (painful arc).
- Check passive abduction.
- Check resisted abduction.
- Check resisted lateral rotation.
- Check resisted medial rotation.

**TABLE 5.7** OSCE marking criteria for physical examination of the shoulder

| MARKING CRITERIA – PHYSICAL EXAMINATION OF THE SHOULDER |
| --- |

Student shows warm approach to patient

Student explains examination procedure to patient

Student exposes area fully prior to performing examination

Student mentions observation of pain when the patient is undressing

Student inspects the patient's neck, noting any abnormalities

Student inspects in a systematic fashion, anterior, posterior, and lateral aspects of both shoulders for
- shape
- symmetry
- visible swellings
- deformity
- redness
- muscle wasting
- scars and/or skin lesions

Student palpates neck muscles (sternomastoid, trapezius) for tenderness, swelling, lumps

Student palpates both shoulders in a systematic fashion for warmth, tenderness, swelling, lumps and muscle bulk (elicits site of pain prior to examination and palpates painful area last) and specifically assesses
- sternoclavicular joint
- clavicle
- acromioclavicular joint
- subacromial and sub-deltoid bursae
- tuberosity of humerus/glenohumeral joint
- bicipital groove and tendon
- biceps
- deltoid
- triceps

Student checks both shoulders for signs of instability
- anterior
- posterior
- inferior

Student assess neurovascular sensation in both arms
- axillary (badge sign)
- radial
- ulna
- median

Student checks neck movements
- flexion
- extension
- lateral bending/flexion
- rotation

(*continued*)

---

**MARKING CRITERIA – PHYSICAL EXAMINATION OF THE SHOULDER**

---

Student assesses active range of movement in both shoulders, noting when pain is elicited and/or limitation of movement

- forward flexion
- extension/hyperextension
- internal rotation
- external rotation

Student assess abduction (painful arc) in both arms

- active abduction (integrity of supraspinatus)
- passive abduction (subacromial bursa)

Student assess resisted movements

- resisted abduction (supraspinatus)
- resisted lateral (external) rotation (infraspinatus/teres minor)
- resisted medial (internal) rotation (subscapularis)

---

## Knee musculoskeletal examination

A typical OSCE physical examination scenario for a knee problem is a patient presenting with medial knee pain after a fall or twisting injury to the knee.

Remember the musculoskeletal examination sequence of:

- inspection
- palpation
- movement
- Selected special tests

Before you undertake your OSCE review the anatomy of the knee, particularly its supporting ligaments:

- medial collateral ligament
- lateral collateral ligament
- anterior cruciate ligament
- posterior cruciate ligament
  - medial meniscus
  - lateral meniscus
  - patella
  - patellar ligament
  - quadriceps ligament
  - bursae of the knee

General inspection

Observe patient for any signs of immediate concern/distress such as:

- possible dislocated patella
- an observed inability to bear weight

- an observed inability to flex or extend the knee
- a large, tense effusion occurring within 1–2 hours post-injury
- distal neurovascular deficit
- knee injury in people > 55 years old (requires X-ray).

Knee inspection
- Ensure the patient is adequately exposed. You need to be able to see both knees, the pelvis and the lower legs/feet.
- Inspect and compare both knees.
- Ideally observe the patient's knee while they are walking, standing, sitting and supine.
- When the patient is standing does the pelvis appear level? The knees should appear symmetrical, anterior/posterior (you can inspect the popliteal fossa area while the patient is standing) and check that the leg lengths are equal when the patient is supine.
- Observe for swelling, erythema and scars or wounds.
- Ask the patient to indicate their perceived area of knee pain.

Knee palpation
Systematically palpate in turn:
- quadriceps/quadriceps ligament and tendon
- patella/patellar ligament/prepatellar bursae
- check for small effusions with a patellar tap test (press down on patella and compare with the unaffected side, looking for spongy resistance, which may indicate a small effusion)
- medial/lateral femoral epicondyles
- medial/lateral menisci
- collateral ligaments
- biceps femoris (hamstring)
- gastrocnemius
- popliteal fossa – nodes/artery
- semi-membranous muscle
- gastrocnemius/semi-membranous bursae.

Knee movements:
- flexion
- extension/hyperextension
- straight leg raising (if the patient is unable to straight leg raise from the bed, lift up the patient's foot and ask them to straight leg raise again. Most people will be able to do so then)

- resistance flexion
- resistance extension.

### Selected special tests – knee

A large range of special tests for the knee are available, many of which are used solely by knee specialists. Presented below is a selected range of knee tests that are simple to perform and test all the major problem areas commonly found in the knee (collateral ligaments, cruciate ligaments and menisci).

Special test 1 – valgus stress test
The valgus stress test assesses the integrity of the medial collateral ligament.
- Ask the patient to lie supine and test the knee in extension and flexed to 15–20°.
- Push the knee medially with one hand while applying an opposing lateral force at the ankle with other hand.
- With the knee in extension, medial collateral ligament instability is felt as a laxity and separation of the tibia and femur (this occurs only in a major disruption of the medial collateral ligament).
- With the knee in flexion, this isolates the medial collateral ligament. You are looking for increased laxity in comparison with the unaffected side and pain on the medial aspect of the knee.

Special test 2 – varus stress test
- The varus stress test assesses the integrity of the lateral collateral ligament. It is the opposite manoeuvre to the valgus stress test.
- Push the knee laterally with one hand while applying an opposing medial force at the ankle with other hand.
- You are looking for increased laxity in comparison with the unaffected side and pain on the lateral aspect of the knee.

Special test 3 – anterior and posterior drawer tests
- For anterior cruciate ligament, you can use the anterior drawer test, where the patient is supine with the knee flexed to 90°.
- Grasp their tibia just below the joint line and pull forward with both your hands.
- An intact anterior cruciate ligament will move forward by only a few millimetres and then stop abruptly with a hard end point and no pain.
- An injured anterior cruciate ligament will have more forward movement and a 'soft' end point, with accompanying pain.

- You can perform an opposite backward movement to check the posterior cruciate ligament (posterior drawer test).

Alternative special test 3 – Lachman's
This is an alternative special test to the anterior drawer test. Lachman's test can sometimes be more sensitive for identifying injury to the anterior cruciate ligament than the drawer test.
- Ask the patient to lie supine, place their knee flexed to 20–30° and pull forward on the proximal tibia, while stabilising the distal femur.
- Abnormal forward motion of the tibia or a soft end feel, often accompanied by pain, is a positive test.
- Compare the affected knee with the unaffected side.

Special test 4 – Apley's grinding test
Apley's grinding test is used to determine if the knee joint line pain is either meniscal or ligamentous.
- Ask the patient to lie prone, with their knee flexed to 90°. Rotate their tibia externally and internally while applying a downward force. Pain at the joint is suggestive of meniscal damage.
- You can then repeat the tibial external/internal rotation using an *upward* force. Pain at this point is suggestive of ligamentous injury.

Alternative special test 4 – McMurray's test
This is an alternative special test to Apley's grinding test.
- Ask the patient to lie supine with their knee maximally flexed.
- Place your fingers on the medial or lateral joint line, and slowly extend the knee with the tibia externally rotated for medial meniscus or internally rotated for the lateral meniscus.
- The test is positive if painful clicking occurs at medial or lateral joint line.

---

**Summary sequence for knee musculoskeletal examination**
- General inspection
- Observe the patient's gait
- Inspect the patient's knees
- Palpate the patient's knees
- Check the knee movements: active straight leg raising extension/flexion, resistance extension/flexion
- Perform the valgus stress test (medial collateral ligament)
- Perform the varus stress test (lateral collateral ligament)

---

○ Perform the anterior drawer test *or* Lachman's (anterior cruciate ligament)
○ Perform the posterior drawer test (posterior cruciate ligament)
○ Perform Apley grinding test or McMurray's (menisci).

**TABLE 5.8** OSCE marking criteria for physical examination of the knee

| MARKING CRITERIA – PHYSICAL EXAMINATION OF THE KNEE |
| --- |
| Student shows a warm overall approach to patient |
| Student asks patient to walk around room |
| Student ensures adequate exposure of both knees/legs |
| Student inspects both knees/legs with patient on bed |
| Student palpates affected knee checking for localised tenderness |
| Student palpates affected knee checking for an effusion using<br>• bulge test or<br>• patellar tap |
| Student asks patient to actively straight leg raise |
| Student checks range of movement of both knees<br>• active – flexion and extension<br>• resistance movements – flexion and extension |
| Student tests stability of both knees by testing collateral ligaments:<br>• medial collateral ligament – valgus stress test<br>• lateral collateral ligament – varus stress test |
| Student tests stability of both knees by testing cruciate ligaments<br>• anterior cruciate ligament using anterior drawer test *or* Lachman's test<br>• posterior cruciate ligament using posterior drawer test |
| Student tests stability of both knees by testing menisci using<br>• Apley's grinding test or<br>• McMurray's test |

## Neurological examination

The completion of a head-to-toe neurological examination encompassing all 12 CNs can be a daunting process for many students, and the time limits of a typical OSCE often prohibit the inclusion of such a full examination. Accordingly, an OSCE neurological physical examination often comprises a focused scenario that requires the student to select components of the full neurological examination as necessitated by the patient's presentation. Examples of a focused neurological OSCE scenario include a patient presenting with a headache or a patient presenting with symptoms of a transient ischaemic attack.

Detailed below is firstly, testing of the 12 CNs, and secondly, the other components of neurological examination such as inspection, locomotor testing and sensation testing.

## Cognitive assessment

A cognitive assesment includes the following:
- appearance and behaviour of the patient
- the patient's speech and language
- the patient's mood
- the patient's thoughts and perceptions
- the patient's cognitive function (memory, attention, information and vocabulary, calculation); the mini-mental state examination is an example of a cognitive function test).

## CN testing

### CN I – olfactory

This is a sensory nerve conveying the sense of smell.
- Ask if the patient has noted any changes in their sense of smell.
- Check the patency of each nostril by asking the patient to sniff.
- Test the ability to smell in each nostril separately, using a sniff test (for example, vanilla essence or coffee granules).

### CN II – optic nerve

This is a sensory nerve conveying the sense of vision from the retina.
- Check visual acuity using a Snellen chart.
- Check visual fields by testing alternate eyes (sometimes called confrontation).
- Test the left visual field. Sit or stand approx 1–2 m opposite the patient with your eyes at the same level as the patient's. Ask the patient to cover their right eye with their right hand. Cover your left eye with your left hand. Ask the patient to look at your uncovered eye with their uncovered eye. Hold your free hand at arm's length equidistant from you and the patient and move it or a held object (such as a pen) into the two temporal quadrants (upper/lower) and then swap your hands over to test the two nasal quadrants (upper/lower). On each occasion ask the patient to say immediately when they can see your hand or the held object. Covering your eye enables you to use your visual fields as a comparative check.
- Check the direct and consensual pupil reactions.
- Undertake a fundoscopy, or be prepared to describe the process of fundoscopy.

- To start fundoscopy set the ophthalmoscope to the '0' dioptre, select the medium-sized round light and shine the light at the patient's pupil while you look down the ophthalmoscope lens in order to elicit the red light reflex. Remember that the optic disc is located on the nasal side of the eye and should normally be a pale orange colour with sharp margins.

### CNs III, IV, VI – oculomotor, trochlear and abducens
These CNs are considered together as they supply the extraocular muscles.
- Inspect and observe eyelids for symmetry and ptosis.
- Inspect and observe the pupil size and symmetry and test for direct and consensual response.
- Check the ocular movements, including the cardinal positions of gaze (patient's eyes following an H pattern in the air) and convergence, and note any sustained beats of nystagmus.

### CN V – trigeminal nerve
This nerve is divided into three branches, ophthalmic, maxillary and mandibular.
- Check the motor component – equality and muscle strength of masseter and also temporal muscles. Also ask patient to open their jaw against resistance.
- Observe for signs of facial muscle wasting.
- Check the sensory component – test over the three divisions, the forehead (ophthalmic), the cheeks (maxillary) and the chin (mandibular).
- Check the corneal reflex – touch the cornea with a cotton wool wisp and observe for blinking.

### CN VII – facial nerve
- Check the muscles of facial expression – observe the face for asymmetry, facial expression and involuntary muscular movements.
- Check for equality and symmetry of muscle strength – ask the patient to smile/bare their teeth, puff out their cheeks, screw up eyes, frowning, and raise eyebrows.

### CN VIII – vestibulocochlear nerve (acoustic)
Sensory nerve with two functions:
- auditory – hearing
- labyrinthine – balance.

Auditory testing includes the whisper test, the Rinne test and the Weber test.
Whisper test:

- Ask patient to occlude one ear.
- Stand behind the patient and whisper '94' or similar, increase the intensity until patient can hear. Repeat for other ear.

The Weber tuning fork test

- Place the base of the small tuning fork (512 hz) firmly on top of the patient's head or on their mid forehead.
- Ask patient where they hear it – on one or on both sides.
- Normal hearing is equal on both sides.

The Rinne tuning fork test (a comparison of air and bone conduction)

- Place a lightly vibrating tuning fork on the mastoid bone.
- Ask the patient to say when they can no longer hear it, then quickly place it close to the ear.
- Normal – air conduction lasts longer than bone conduction.

### CN IX – glossopharyngeal and CN X – vagus nerve

- Observe whether the patient's speech is clear.
- Ask the patient to say 'Aah' and observe their soft palate movement (phonation).
- If needed elicit the pharyngeal (gag) reflex by gently touching the posterior pharynx with a tongue depressor.

### CN XI – spinal accessory (previously seen in neck and back examination)

The motor nerve supplying the sternocleidomastoid and trapezius muscles.

- Sternocleidomastoid – ask the patient to turn their head to either side against resistance.
- Trapezius – ask the patient to shrug shoulders against resistance.

### CN XII – hypoglossal

This is a motor nerve supplying the tongue.

- Listen to the patient for clear articulation.
- Inspect the tongue for atrophy and fasciculation.
- With the patient's tongue protruded, look for asymmetry and medial deviation.
- Ask the patient to move their tongue from side to side.
- Check the tongue strength (push tongue against cheek).

## A mnemonic device to help remember the names of the CNs

| | | | |
|---|---|---|---|
| ○ CNI | **O**lfactory | **O**n |
| ○ CNII | **O**ptic | **O**ld |
| ○ CNIII | **O**culomotor | **O**lympus |
| ○ CNIV | **T**rochlear | **T**owering |
| ○ CNV | **T**rigeminal | **T**ops |
| ○ CNVI | **A**bducens | **A**re |
| ○ CNVII | **F**acial | **F**rench |
| ○ CNVIII | **A**coustic | **A**nd |
| ○ CNIX | **G**lossopharyngeal | **G**erman |
| ○ CNX | **V**agus | **V**ines |
| ○ CNXI | **A**ccessory | **A**nd |
| ○ CNXII | **H**ypoglossal | **H**ops |

**TABLE 5.9** Summary table of CN functions, symptoms and testing

| CN | MAIN FUNCTIONS | SYMPTOMS/SIGNS OF DAMAGE | HOW TO TEST |
|---|---|---|---|
| Olfactory (CN I) | Smell | Altered smell | Sniff test |
| Optic (CN II) | Vision | Visual disturbances Pupil abnormalities | Visual acuity and colour. Visual fields fundoscopy pupils |
| Oculomotor (CN III) | Pupil constriction Opening the eye Extraocular movements | Pupil abnormalities Deviations of the eye Nystagmus Ptosis | Symmetry and eye opening, ptosis, extraocular movements (down and out). Pupils, equal, round, and reactive to light |
| Trochlear (CN IV) | Downward, inward eye movements | Deviations of the eye Nystagmus | Extraocular movements (down and in) |
| Trigeminal (CN V) | *Motor* temporal/ masseter muscles, jaw lateral movement *Sensory* ophthalmic, maxillary, mandibular | Weak masseter/ temporal muscles Decreased facial sensations Absence of blinking | Ophthalmic, maxillary, mandibular test sensation. *Optic* corneal reflex, post ⅓ tongue taste Masseter muscles: resistance to jaw opening, lateral jaw strength |
| Abducens (CN VI) | Lateral deviation of the eye | Deviations of the eye Nystagmus | Extraocular movements lateral movement |

(*continued*)

| CN | MAIN FUNCTIONS | SYMPTOMS/SIGNS OF DAMAGE | HOW TO TEST |
|---|---|---|---|
| Facial (CN VII) | *Motor* facial movements, including expression, eye and mouth closing *Sensory* taste anterior tongue | Drooping of lower eyelid Unilateral facial paralysis Incomplete eyelid closure Impaired blinking | Face at rest, frown, screw up eyes, show teeth and puff out cheeks *Taste* anterior ⅔ tongue |
| Vestibulocochlear (CN VIII) | Hearing and balance | Decreased hearing | Hearing, Rinne, Weber |
| Glossopharyngeal (CN IX) | *Motor* pharynx *Sensory* eardrum, ear canal, pharynx, taste posterior tongue | Hoarseness Pharynx or palate weakness Asymmetrical palate rising Decreased gag reflex | Bitter taste posterior ⅓ Gag reflex symmetrical rise of pharynx |
| Vagus (CN X) | *Motor* palate, pharynx, larynx *Sensory* pharynx and larynx | Hoarseness Pharynx or palate weakness Asymmetrical palate rising Decreased gag reflex | Sensation pharynx and larynx Movement of uvula and position, swallow, speech |
| Spinal accessory (CN XI) | *Motor* sternocleidomastoid and upper position of trapezius | Muscle weakness Asymmetry of shoulders | Trapezius – shoulder shrug against resistance Sternocleidomastoid – face turned against resistance |
| Hypoglossal (CN XII) | *Motor* tongue | Poor articulation Impaired tongue movements Deviated tongue | Tongue symmetry, fasciculation and strength |

## Neurological inspection

Observe the patient for:

- posture, gait, co-ordination, abnormal movements
- wasting – note symmetry and distribution (proximal wasting)
- fasciculation – spontaneous contraction of muscle areas
- tremors.

## Neurological palpation

Palpate the muscle groups of the body, noting:

- muscle bulk – look for atrophy of the hands, shoulders and thighs
- muscular tenderness.

### Assessment of muscular tone

Normal muscles with intact nerve supplies maintain a slight residual tension known as muscle tone. Patient should be relaxed and lying in a neutral position. There is normally limited resistance through a range of movements Check for:

- hypertonia – resistance then release (Parkinson's disease)
- hypotonia – (marked floppiness) due to lower motor neuron or cerebellar lesions.

### Assessment of muscle strength

Check all muscle groups against resistance:

- neck rotation to right and left
- shoulder abduction and adduction
- elbow flexion (C5, C6) extension (C6, C7, C8). Patient pushes and pulls against your hand
- wrist extension (C6, C7, C8, radial nerve). Patient makes a fist and resists you pulling it down
- grip (C7, C8, T1). The patient squeezes two of your fingers as hard as they can
- finger abduction (C8, T1, ulnar nerve). The patient's hand is spread with palm down. Ask patient to resist as you try to force their fingers together
- thumb opposition (C8, T1, median nerve). The patient tries to touch little finger to thumb against your resistance
- hip flexion (L2, L3, L4). Place hand on the patient's thighs and ask them to raise their leg against hand
- hip adduction (L2, L3, L4). Place your hand between the patient's knees and ask them to bring both legs together
- hip abduction (14, L5, S1). Place hands outside the patient's knees and ask them to spread legs against your hands
- hip extension (S1). Ask the patient to push posterior thigh against your hand
- knee extension (L2, L3, L4). Support the patient's knee in flexion and ask them to straighten leg
- knee flexion (L4, L5, S1, S2) With the patient's leg in flexion and foot on the bed ask the patient to keep the foot down as you straighten the leg
- ankle dorsiflexion (L4, L5). Ask the patient to pull and push against your hand
- ankle plantar flexion (S1). Ask the patient to pull and push against your hand.

### Reflexes
Check the following reflexes:
- brachioradialis (supinator) (C5, C6), direct 2.5–5 cm above wrist (flexion and supination)
- biceps (C5, C6), indirect at antecubital space (elbow flexion and biceps contraction)
- triceps (C6, C7), direct, above elbow (elbow extension and triceps contraction)
- knee (L2, L3, L4), direct at insertion of patella tendon (knee extension and quadriceps contraction)
- ankle (S1), direct, above heel (plantar flexion at the ankle)
- plantar (L5, S1), direct from heel to toes (movement of toes normally plantar flexion).

### Co-ordination
Ask the patient to perform the following:
- rapid alternating movements (hands and feet)
- point-to-point movements (nose to finger and heal to shin bilaterally)
- hop on alternate legs and shallow knee bends.

### Gait
- Ask the patient to walk across the room and observe if their gait is smooth and co-ordinated.
- A gait that lacks co-ordination is called ataxic; this may be due to cerebella dysfunction, loss of position sense or alcohol or drug intoxication.
- Then assess tandem gait (walking heel to toe) – this may reveal ataxia not previously obvious.
- Ask the patient to walk on their heels and then toes – this may indicate muscle weakness.

### Sensory
- Pin (using a monofilament) – superficial pain is elicited.
- Light touch – use wisps of cotton wool.
- Test in this suggested pattern starting with shoulders (C4), forearms (C6/T1), thumbs and little fingers (C6/C8), anterior thighs (L2), lateral and medial calves (L4/L5), little toes (S1), medial buttocks (S3).
- Vibration sensitivity – use large 128 Hz tuning fork at distal joints – often the first sense to be decreased in peripheral neuropathy.
- Position sense – hold both sides of fingers and toes to elicit up or down movements while the patient is looking away or has their eyes closed

– loss of position sense may indicate a central lesion or a lesion of peripheral nerve or root.

- Discrimination – ask the patient to identify a small object placed in each hand, one at a time. If touch and position sense are normal, this can usually be done. An inability to discriminate may suggest a disease of the sensory cortex.
- Romberg test – Ask patient to stand upright with feet together and their eyes closed. A positive test is when the patient is steady with eyes open, but feels off balance or is unsteady with eyes closed (a slight wobble can be normal).

---

### Summary sequence for neurological examination

- Cognitive assessment
- CN I (smell)
- CN II acuity, visual fields, pupils, fundoscopy
- CN III, IV and VI eyelid symmetry, pupils, eye movements
- CN V facial sensations, motor, corneal reflex
- CN VII facial expression, asymmetry, facial movements
- CN VIII whisper test, tuning fork tests
- CN IX, X taste, gag reflex, palate rise on phonation, hoarse voice
- CN XI turn face against resistance, shoulder shrug
- CN XII articulation, abnormal tongue movements, tongue symmetry and movement, tongue strength
- Motor function inspection, palpation, muscle tone, muscle power, tendon reflexes, co-ordination, check gait
- Sensory system light touch, pin prick, vibration, joint position sense, discrimination, Romberg test.

---

**TABLE 5.10** OSCE marking criteria for a patient presenting with symptoms suggestive of a transient ischaemic attack

Due to the number of components to be completed this OSCE would normally be longer than a 10 minute station

| MARKING CRITERIA – A TRANSIENT ISCHAEMIC ATTACK |
| --- |
| Student obtains patient's consent and explains the examination |
| Student exposes patient appropriately for each element of physical examination |
| Student performs general observation of patient |
| Student assesses the patient's orientation to time, place and person |

(continued)

### MARKING CRITERIA – A TRANSIENT ISCHAEMIC ATTACK

Student says they would do base line observations of temperature, BP, pulse and respirations

Student listens for carotid bruits to assess possible carotid blockage

Student assesses appropriate CNs bilaterally

#### CN 2 – optic nerve – visual acuity

Student performs optic fundoscopy on one eye only and describes the process, e.g. would identify red reflex, vessels, optic disc, retina

Student assesses the patient's visual fields (by confrontation)

Student assesses the patient's pupil reaction to light (direct and consensual response)

Student assesses accommodation

#### CNs 3, 4, 6 – oculomotor, trochlear and abducens

Student checks six cardinal positions of gaze

Student checks for convergence

Student looks for ptosis (drooping of the upper eye lid)

#### Student checks CN 5 – trigeminal

Sensation (optic, maxillary, mandible)

Student checks motor (jaw clench, open jaw, side to side)

#### Student checks CN 7 – facial

Facial movements (frown, puff out cheeks, raises eyebrows etc.)

#### Student checks CN 8 – cochlea vestibular

Notes whether gross hearing is intact (whisper test)

#### Student checks CNs 9 and 10 – glossopharyneal and vagus

Student listen to patient's voice

Student asks the patient if they have any difficulty in swallowing

Student asks the patient to say, 'Aah'

Student says they will test the gag reflex

#### Student checks CN 11 – spinal accessory

Motor (shoulder shrug and neck strength)

#### Student checks CN 12 – hypoglossal

Student listens to the articulation of the patient's words

Student inspects the patient's tongue, looking for atrophy or fasciculation

Student asks patient to stick out tongue

Student asks patient to move tongue from side to side

Student checks for tongue strength

Student assesses motor function of upper limbs

Observes upper body position

Student compares size and contours of upper body muscles

Student assesses muscle tone and tests for muscle strength
- abduction and adduction of shoulders bilaterally
- flexion and extension of the elbows bilaterally
- extension of the wrist

*(continued)*

---

**MARKING CRITERIA – A TRANSIENT ISCHAEMIC ATTACK**

---

Student assesses muscle tone and tests for muscle strength (cont.)

- handgrip – bilaterally
- finger abduction – bilaterally
- thumb opposition

Student assesses co-ordination

Looks at patient's gait and asks the patient to

- walk heel to toe (tandem walk)
- walk on their toes
- walk on their heels
- hop on one leg then the other
- perform a shallow knee bend or asks patient to rise from a sitting position without arm support
- perform the Romberg test – and notes the patient's ability to maintain an upright position

Student assesses for pronator drift

Student assesses for rapid alternating movements of the hands and feet

Student assesses for point-to-point movements of arms and legs

Student assesses the sensory system

Assesses for pain using 'sharp or dull' in appropriate places on the body, arms and legs

Student assesses for light touch as appropriate

Student assesses for discrimination using stereognosis

Student tests reflexes in upper limbs

- the biceps tendon
- the triceps tendon
- brachioradialis tendon

Student tests reflexes in lower limbs

- knee reflex
- Achilles reflex
- plantar reflex

---

## An example of an abbreviated neurological examination for a patient presenting with a headache

This brief neurological exam uses selected components of the full neurological examination, and is an example of selectively applying neurological examination techniques in relation to a patient's presenting problem; in this case for OSCE patients whose history suggests a migraine or tension-type headache (adapted from 'A 3 minute neurological examination for use in recurrent headache').[1]

1  **Romberg's test** – most people wobble: look for falling or swaying.
2  **Tandem gait** – may be more difficult to complete than the Romberg test.
3  **Walking on heels** – tests the power of ankle dorsiflexion.

4 **Outstretched arms** – with upturned palms and eyes closed: look for pronation and drift of arms.

5 **Finger–nose test** – with eyes closed, tests light touch and co-ordination. You can observe pupil response when the patient opens their eyes (accommodation).

6 **Fine finger movements** – of both hands: the patient should move each finger independently.

7 **Finger taps** – for both hands, should be rapid.

8 **Visual fields** – alternate eye testing of upper and lower temporal and nasal fields.

9 **Eye movements** – look for sustained nystagmus and/or jerky eye movements.

10 **Face and tongue movements** – ask patient to screw up their eyes, smile widely and stick out their tongue.

11 **Fundoscopy** – first check pupil reactions, and then looking for papilloedema (this is rare in people who are alert and orientated).

12 **Reflexes and plantars** – brisk responses are significant only if accompanied by muscle weakness or increased tone or extensor plantar response. Diminished reflexes are rarely relevant in patients presenting with simple headaches.

## Paediatric physical examination

As with history taking stations, you may sometimes be asked to undertake a physical examination station for a child, even if you are not taking a paediatric-focused course. This is because many nurse practitioner students will potentially be working in areas where contact with children would occur, such as in primary healthcare. As with paediatric history taking stations, physical examination stations do not normally use a child as the actual patient, but instead use someone playing the role of the carer and an age-appropriate child-sized mannequin in place of a child. Remember that this is a role-playing situation and you should attempt to interact with the carer and mannequin as you would do normally in clinical practice in order to demonstrate your ability to apply your paediatric physical examination skills.

Common scenarios that may be used for a paediatric physical examination station include a child presenting with a fever, a child presenting with a rash, and a child presenting with diarrhoea and vomiting. Please note that unless you are undertaking a paediatric-focused course, most paediatric OSCE scenarios would use a child in the age range from 2 years old and above.

In contrast to problem-focused adult physical examination, paediatric physical examination typically requires a top-to-toe approach to ensure a sufficiently comprehensive examination. The following is an example of a top-to-toe sequence.

- A general inspection and ensuring that the child mannequin's clothing is appropriately removed for the examination.
- Inspection of vital signs including respiratory rate, pulse, temperature and capillary refill time (you would need to be able to interpret these against the normal paediatric values for the age range of your patient).
- Perform an ear, nose and throat examination including the patient's mouth, throat, nose, ears and neck glands.
- Perform a respiratory chest examination, including inspection and auscultation.
- Perform an abdominal examination, including inspection, auscultation and palpation.
- Perform skin inspection and palpation, including an assessment of peripheral perfusion.
- Check for red flag symptoms, such as signs of dehydration (mucous membranes and skin turgor) and also meningitis (light sensitivity and neck stiffness).

**TABLE 5.11** OSCE marking criteria for a 3-year-old child presenting with a rash

| MARKING CRITERIA – A 3-YEAR-OLD CHILD PRESENTING WITH A RASH |
| --- |
| Student introduces self to child and attempts to put the child at ease, using appropriate distraction |
| Student explains what they are doing, appropriate to age and developmental stage of child |
| Student asks the carer to undress the child, ensuring that the child is adequately exposed |
| Student washes their hands |
| Student observes the general condition of child (alert, interactive, playful, irritable, lethargic) |
| Student takes vital signs<br>• temperature<br>• pulse<br>• respiratory rate<br>• capillary refill time<br>Student compares vital signs to age-appropriate values |
| **Physical examination** |
| Student inspects skin for<br>• colour<br>• rash/lesions – distribution, morphology, pattern |

(*continued*)

MARKING CRITERIA – A 3-YEAR-OLD CHILD PRESENTING WITH A RASH

**Red flag – Hydration**
Student checks moisture of mouth
Checks skin turgor

**Respiratory examination**
Student inspects the chest for
- respiratory distress
- use of accessory muscles
- recession
- chest shape

Student auscultates using correct technique (one full inspiratory/expiratory cycle)
Student checks four places on anterior chest
Student checks four places on posterior chest
Student explains what they are listening for (air entry, added sounds, e.g. crackles, wheezes)

**ENT examination**
Student instructs carer on appropriate restraint during the examination
Student examines ears using age-appropriate technique and explains what they are looking for
Student examines the patient's throat and explains what they are looking for
Student examines the lymph nodes of head and neck

**Eyes**
Student examines the patient's eyes for
- discharge
- redness

**Red flag – signs of meningitis**
Student examines for photophobia
Student checks for neck stiffness

**Abdomen**
Student inspects for swelling, distension
Student auscultates for bowel sounds
Student palpates for softness, rigidity, guarding, tenderness

**Peripheries**
Student checks for warmth/perfusion

---

## Physical examination OSCE stations in summary

As with the related clinical skill of history taking, the key to success in OSCE physical examination is **practising**; whether this is in your clinical setting, with student colleagues, or with friends and family. You must also ensure that you commit to memory the summary examination sequences for each of the body systems, as detailed above. In general, the following seven-step summary sequence can be used to structure your performance at physical examination OSCE stations:

○ Introduce yourself.
○ Confirm with the patient the type of examination sequence you need to undertake and obtain their consent.
○ Perform a general inspection and observe the vital signs.
○ Perform a specific inspection of patient's problem area (diagnostic equipment may need to be used for this).
○ Perform palpation as required.
○ Perform percussion (if required).
○ Perform auscultation (if required).
○ Finally, please remember that during an OSCE physical examination station you need to actually examine the patient, rather than just talk about examining them.

## Reference

1 Anonymous author. *A three minute neurological examination for use in recurrent headache.* Reference number 97/7362. Wilmslow: Zeneca Pharma; 1997.

## Further reading

Bickley L, Szilagyi P. *Bates' Guide to Physical Examination and History Taking.* 9th ed. London: Lippincott; 2007.

Cross S, Rimmer M, editors. *Nurse Practitioner Manual of Clinical Skills.* 2nd ed. Edinburgh: Bailliere Tindall; 2007.

Thomas J, Monaghan T, editors. *Oxford Handbook of Clinical Examination and Practical Skills.* Oxford: Oxford University Press; 2007.

Walsh M, Crumbie A, Reveley S, editors. *Nurse Practitioners: Clinical Skills and Professional Issues.* 2nd ed. Oxford: Butterworth Heinemann; 2006.

# 6

# Question and answer OSCE stations

### The purpose of question and answer stations

The OSCE question and answer station format has been developed by the advanced nursing team at London South Bank University as an alternative to a traditional written examination, as we have found that students are often able to express themselves more accurately verbally than in a written response in a traditional unseen, paper-based exam. OSCE question and answer stations lend themselves to scenarios that would be otherwise very difficult to role-play, for example, a paediatric scenario (as children are not normally used in OSCEs), an urgent situation (such as patient presenting with cardiac chest pain or a severe allergic reaction) or a sexual health scenario (due to the intimate nature of these presentations). Question and answer OSCE stations are normally designed to ensure that the questions are clear and not at all ambiguous. The questions need be understood fully; therefore short concise questions are better than long complex questions. For example:

**Question:** List the red flag signs and symptoms of meningitis

**▶❗ Answer:**
- a high fever that does not resolve with antipyretic medication
- a stiff neck
- non-blanching rash
- photophobia
- a positive Kernig's (bilateral posterior knee pain occurring on passive extension of the knees)

- irritability
- increased drowsiness/decreased consciousness
- fits
- vomiting
- tachycardia/bradycardia
- raised blood pressure
- bulging fontanelle (infant)
- abnormal tone/posture
- decreased peripheral perfusion
- tachypnoea (rapid shallow breathing).

All the possible signs and symptoms must be documented and the examiner must interpret the answer as accurately as possible, for example if the student uses a lay term rather than medical terminology the answer would still be correct. The scoring system must be clear and essential red flag answers must be addressed by the student. In the above example, a student must answer 10/15 points correctly to pass the question, including the red flags such as photophobia, non-blanching rash, neck stiffness and unresponsive fever.

Questions such as 'What would you do next?' are useful for assessing the student's ability to act in an urgent situation. For example:

*Question:* Mrs Green, a 65-year-old women, becomes acutely unwell with dyspnoea and possible angio-oedema following the administration of the 'flu vaccine. What would you do next?

*Answer:*
- call for help
- dial 999
- observe blood pressure and pulse
- ensure patient is comfortable on a flat surface, such as an exam couch
- give oxygen
- give adrenaline (epinephrine) injection.

The student would need to give 4/6 actions to pass the above question, including help/assistance, oxygen and adrenaline administration.

Questions to assess the student's clinical reasoning can also be used in a question and answer station. This is particularly useful as shorter (5 or 10 minute) OSCE stations may not lend themselves to the assessment of clinical reasoning skills. For example: given the following scenario, list six possible multiple hypotheses.

*Scenario*: Mr Patel is a 65-year-old Asian patient presenting with acute onset of chest pain and shortness of breath. He has a past medical history of hypertension and type 2 diabetes. He has just returned from India.

*Examples of possible answers:*
- myocardial infarction
- angina
- pulmonary embolism
- heart failure
- pneumothorax
- chest infection
- acute asthma attack
- exacerbation of chronic obstructive pulmonary disease.

Question and answer stations may also lend themselves to questions around health promotion or the treatment and management of a specific scenario. For example:

*Question*: What advice would you give Mr Patel following his diagnosis of angina?

*Answer:*
- stop smoking (if appropriate)
- dietary advice – change to a low fat, low salt, less red meat, low sugar diet
- alcohol advice (if appropriate)
- stress management
- weight loss programme
- exercise programme
- how to take prescribed medication, e.g. angina spray
- what to do if he experiences the pain again
- when to call for an ambulance.

In the above example the student must provide 6/9 examples of advice (including advice on stopping smoking)

## How to respond to question and answer stations

You should practise question and answer stations beforehand to ensure that you are familiar with the format. If you do not immediately understand the question, ask the examiner to repeat it. Do not be afraid to repeat yourself, it is better to say something twice than not at all. If you lose track of what you have said, summarise the answer, as this can be a useful method for recalling the question.

Try not to forget the obvious. For example, if you are asked what physical examination procedure you need to undertake, do not forget to include baseline observations of temperature, pulse, blood pressure and respirations: they will all carry marks.

Ensure that you answer the question in a logical order, for example, if the question is 'What would you do next?' think about the order in which you would do the procedure in your own clinical area.

Try to use correct medical/nursing terminology, as you are talking to an examiner not a patient. This would be your opportunity to demonstrate that you have a good understanding of specific medical terminologies.

Revise the red flags for a range of urgent scenarios, such as chest pain, acute dyspnoea, child fever, allergic reactions and asthma exacerbations. You should also revise the treatment and management for these types of urgent scenarios.

Do not look to the examiner for clues, as you may misinterpret their non-verbal communication. Remember that at a question and answer station the examiner merely ticks off your answers on the exam paper, while the other person does not play the role of patient, but instead asks you the question that you need to answer.

## Sample question and answer OSCE stations
### Childhood asthma exacerbation question and answer station

'Sally is a 7-year-old child who has been brought in by her father to your same-day/urgent session with an exacerbation of her asthma.'

*Question 1 What immediate physical signs would you look for when you meet Sally on her arrival?*

| CRITERIA | MENTIONED | NOT MENTIONED |
|---|---|---|
| Assess level of distress/agitation | | |
| *Assess colour for cyanosis | | |
| Assess for audible wheeze | | |
| Can she complete a sentence in one breath? | | |
| Assess for use of accessory muscles (neck) | | |
| Is she coughing? | | |

*(continued)*

| CRITERIA | MENTIONED | NOT MENTIONED |
|---|---|---|
| Is she short of breath? | | |
| Is she exhausted? | | |
| *Assess consciousness level. Is she drowsy? | | |

Marking criteria: 5 out of 9 (must include*)

### Question 2 Which aspects of history do you need to get from Sally's father?

| CRITERIA | MENTIONED | NOT MENTIONED |
|---|---|---|
| Time of onset of attack | | |
| *Was it gradual or acute onset? | | |
| *How has she been treated so far? | | |
| *Has there been any relief? | | |
| Has she a history of severe asthma attacks/ hospital admissions? | | |
| How is her asthma normally managed? | | |
| Does she comply with the medicines? | | |
| Has there been any change in Sally's asthma medication or delivery device? | | |
| Have you noticed an increase in her use of reliever medication recently? | | |
| Does Sally have any other medical problems, such as a recent respiratory tract infection? | | |
| Does she have a cough? | | |
| If so, when does it occur? Nocturnal? Productive? | | |
| Is she short of breath on exertion? | | |
| Is she taking any new or other medications – including over-the-counter medication? | | |
| Has she been in contact with any triggers, e.g. pets, smoke or other known allergens? | | |
| Have there been any recent events in Sally's life that might have upset her? | | |

Marking criteria: 10 out of 16 (must include*)

## Question 3 *What physical assessment would you like to perform on Sally?*

| CRITERIA | MENTIONED | NOT MENTIONED |
|---|---|---|
| *Baseline observations of respiratory rate | | |
| *Assess degree of breathlessness/too breathless to complete a sentence in one breath | | |
| *Assess pulse/oxygen saturation (if available) | | |
| Check temperature | | |
| Check peak flow compared to personal best or predicted value | | |
| *Check use of accessory muscles of respiration (in neck) | | |
| *Perform full physical examination of the chest Auscultation for wheezes | | |
| *Check air entry/silent chest | | |

Marking criteria: 6 out of 8 (must include*)

## Question 4 *What red flags for asthma you would look for?*

| CRITERIA | MENTIONED | NOT MENTIONED |
|---|---|---|
| *Cyanosis | | |
| Inability to complete a sentence in one breath Or: too breathless to talk or feed | | |
| *Silent chest | | |
| *Pulse rate above 120 | | |
| *Respiratory rate above 30 | | |
| Oxygen saturation < 92% | | |
| Peak flow < 33% predicted | | |
| Use of accessory muscles of respiration | | |
| Poor response to relief medication | | |
| *Weak respiratory effort | | |
| Exhaustion | | |
| Confusion | | |
| Coma | | |
| Previous recent hospital admissions | | |

Marking criteria: 10 out of 14 (must include*)

## Ischaemic chest pain question and answer station

'Mr Bhati is a 59-year-old Asian patient who has just registered at your surgery. He is complaining of chest pain.'

### Question 1  What immediate observations would you make for a patient who complains of chest pain?

| CRITERIA | MENTIONED | NOT MENTIONED |
|---|---|---|
| Breathing | | |
| Circulation | | |
| Observe patient's general appearance | | |
| Skin colour: perfusion | | |
| Vital signs | | |
| Level of distress | | |
| Sweating | | |
| Clammy | | |

Marking criteria: 4 out of 8

### Question 2  What items would you include in your history?

| CRITERIA | MENTIONED | NOT MENTIONED |
|---|---|---|
| Uses framework to elicit history, e.g. OPQRSTU | | |
| Questions include | | |
| • exclusion of chest trauma | | |
| • epigastric pain after eating | | |
| • cough | | |
| • fever | | |
| • exploration of pain | | |
| • associated signs and symptoms | | |
| Past medical history | | |
| Family history | | |
| High blood pressure | | |
| History of diabetes | | |
| Occupation | | |
| Exercise | | |
| Current medications | | |
| Side effects of medications | | |
| When did he last have an angina spray and how effective was it? | | |
| What does the patient think is wrong? | | |

Marking criteria – exploration of pain and or uses OPQRSTU framework

*Question 3 What immediate investigations would be appropriate for Mr Bhati?*

| CRITERIA | MENTIONED | NOT MENTIONED |
|---|---|---|
| Electrocardiogram (if available) | | |
| Oxygen saturation (if available) | | |

Marking criteria: ECG or O$_2$ saturation, depending on their availability

*Question 4 What immediate management would be appropriate for Mr Bhati?*

| CRITERIA | MENTIONED | NOT MENTIONED |
|---|---|---|
| Give oxygen (if available) | | |
| Call for assistance | | |
| Request emergency ambulance and notify hospital, if applicable. | | |
| Administer aspirin, 300 mg stat | | |
| Monitor the patient's condition on couch/trolley until help arrives | | |
| Reassure the patient and keep him as comfortable as possible. | | |
| Liaise with GP/other health professionals if necessary | | |

Marking criteria: minimum is call for help and give aspirin

Mr Bhati has now recovered from a myocardial infarction and been discharged from hospital. He wants to help prevent a further occurrence.

*Question 5 What long-term non-pharmacological management would be appropriate for Mr Bhati?*

| CRITERIA | MENTIONED | NOT MENTIONED |
|---|---|---|
| Patient education to include the nature of the disease | | |
| Reduce risk factors overall | | |
| Alcohol intake | | |
| Physical exertion/exercise | | |
| Diet | | |
| Reduce cholesterol and lipids | | |
| Stop smoking advice, if appropriate | | |
| Resuming employment | | |
| Sexual activities | | |

*(continued)*

| CRITERIA | MENTIONED | NOT MENTIONED |
|---|---|---|
| Stress management | | |
| Psychological support including partner/family, if appropriate | | |

Marking criteria: must discuss 1 out of 2.

---

### Question and answer OSCE stations in summary

Question and answer OSCE stations provide an opportunity for you to demonstrate your competence in the assessment and management of patients presenting with potentially urgent clinical problems. You must remember that question and answer stations are presented as *viva voce* style examinations, and so you should be prepared to use your verbally based clinical reasoning skills, much as you would need to in actual clinical practice when managing a clinically urgent situation.

---

## Further reading

Simon C, O'Reilly K, Proctor R, *et al.*, editors. *Emergencies in Primary Care.* Oxford: Oxford University Press; 2007.

# 7

# OSCE stations that assess communication skills, conveying information and treatment and management

This chapter examines a variety of other OSCE stations that can be developed to ensure face validity of the OSCE, as they can assess areas of the curriculum which may, by their more specialist nature, not be assessed elsewhere in the curriculum.

## Communication skills

An example of this is a station developed to assess students' communication skills in exploring a history that may indicate depression in a patient. Depression is an area that is common both in the primary care setting and in the acute care setting, but is often misdiagnosed or overlooked, due to a lack of insight or inexperience of the clinician taking the history. Students should be aware that approximately 15% of people have an incidence of major depression at some point in their life, and it is the fourth most common cause of disability worldwide;[1] correspondingly, depression assessment is a common OSCE station topic.

A depression-focused OSCE station could use a mental state exam as a framework for the marking criteria or mental health guideline. Use of this type of framework as a marking guideline would not only ensure objectivity, but also enhances the reliability and validity of the station. Broadly, the student is required to ask questions related to the patient's mental health, and as a result of the answers be able to make a diagnosis of mild, moderate or severe depression. It is permissible to use a validated depression rating tool to help structure your questions and determine the severity of the patient's depression.

Depressed patients often lose interest in things that they used to enjoy and their symptoms may interfere with their work or family. Therefore, questions should be centred on these areas, as in the examples below.

The student needs to explore psychological symptoms related to:
- low mood or sadness
- feelings of hopelessness and helplessness
- low self-esteem
- tearfulness
- feelings of guilt
- irritability or intolerance
- lack of motivation or interest
- inability to make decisions
- lack of enjoyment
- suicidal ideation or thoughts of self harm or harming others (red flag)
- feelings of anxiety
- reduced sex drive.

Physical symptoms should also be explored. These include:
- slowed speech or movement
- change in appetite or weight (increased or decreased)
- constipation
- unexplained aches and pains
- lack of energy
- lack of sexual interest
- changes to the menstrual cycle (women).

Social symptoms should be explored, including:
- not performing well at work
- avoiding social activities
- difficulties/changes in home circumstances
- increased use of alcohol/smoking/recreational drugs.

## OSCE for communicating with a depressed patient

'This is Alice, a 34-year-old woman who has presented at your clinic today. You have not met her before.'

Instructions for patient (you should exhibit non-verbal signs of low mood throughout the consultation).

---

**Box 7.1  Scenario for a patient with depression**

You are Alice, a 34-year-old woman who has presented to the nurse practitioner today because you have become increasingly depressed over the last 6 months. You are married with no children. Six months ago you suffered a miscarriage at 12 weeks gestation; this was your first pregnancy. You have a high profile job in the city, nobody at work knows about your pregnancy or miscarriage.

Your husband also works long hours in the city. Your family lives in Scotland and you see them about twice a year. Your husband's family is local, but you don't get on with them on that well. They keep nagging you about starting a family and do not know about the miscarriage.

Both you and your husband were very disappointed about the miscarriage, as you had been trying for a baby for about a year before you became pregnant. Following the miscarriage you have found talking to your husband about it very difficult. Following the miscarriage you have not been interested in sex.

You have found that you are not enjoying your job any more, it is hard to cope with and you are finding it difficult to concentrate. You have not been sleeping very well for the last 6 months and you have found that you wake up very early and cannot go back to sleep.

Your appetite has decreased and you have lost about 4 kg. You have started to drink more wine than you used to (about 4 glasses a night). You have never smoked. You have had no professional support following the miscarriage. You have an overwhelming feeling of guilt/failure as you had the miscarriage following a game of tennis.

Past medical history – nil of note. Family history – nil of note, except your mother suffered with post-natal depression. You have been feeling very low and cry a lot.

If asked directly by the student you should say that you are *not* suicidal, and that you have no other thoughts of self-harm.

---

During your history taking the examiner would be seeing whether you display appropriate empathy and understanding of the patient's problem though your use of effective communication skills. Towards the end of the station you may be asked to provide a provisional diagnosis for the patient's problems, and to comment on any clues you have noted, other than the history taking information, which would support a diagnosis of depression.

**TABLE 7.1** OSCE marking criteria for assessing depression

| MARKING CRITERIA – ASSESSING DEPRESSION |
| --- |

### Part 1

Student introduces self and displays an open, warm approach

Student asks open questions

Student demonstrates listening skills/uses silence appropriately

Student elicits physical symptoms and asks about

- the duration of the current problem
- the patient's sleep pattern
- the patient's appetite/weight changes
- the patient's alcohol consumption
- the patient's smoking
- the patient's miscarriage 6 months ago (after trying for 1 year to become pregnant)
- the patient's lack of interest in sex

Student elicits psychological factors including

- the patient's low mood/sadness
- the patient's feeling of helplessness. hopelessness
- the patient's low self-esteem
- the patient's tearfulness
- the patient's sense of guilt/failure
- the patient's feeling of irritability
- the patient's lack of motivation
- the patient's lack of enjoyment

Student elicits the patient's social symptoms

- the patient's work situation
- the patient's home situation
- the patient's relationship with husband
- the patient's family support
- the patient's past medical history

Student assess the patient's support network

Student elicits the patients ideas/concerns

Student assesses the patient's risk of self-harm/suicide ideation

### Part 2

Student establishes diagnosis – mild depression (post natal/bereavement)

Student observes other signs of depression, such as non-verbal cues, for example, the patient's lack of eye contact, their tone of voice, flat interactions

## Conveying information stations

This type of OSCE station is an ideal way to assess the ability to communicate medical information to a patient in terms that the patient is going to understand rather than in medical or nursing jargon. It could include the interpretation of a laboratory result and then conveying information around a disease process or the treatment and management of the disease related to the laboratory result. An example of this is interpreting a blood test for a lipid profile, treatment options and the subsequent health education around a healthy lifestyle, and the potential consequences of not attempting to lower the lipid profile.

The test results must be realistic for the students who are interpreting them. If the student would normally have a reference range supplied with the test results then this should be supplied, particularly if students come from a geographical spread of clinical settings where the may be slight discrepancies in therapeutic ranges.

Below are two examples of conveying information stations; one for cholesterol, and another one for liver function.

## OSCE station to discuss the results of a cholesterol test

> ### Box 7.2  Patient's cholesterol test results
>
> Patient's name: Mr Jones
> Date of birth: 17 November 1955
> Normal reference range in parentheses
> Total cholesterol: 6.5 mmol (< 5.2 mmol)
> Low-density lipoprotein (LDL) cholesterol (fasting): 4. mmol (< 3.0 mmol)
> High-density lipoprotein (HDL) cholesterol: 1.2 mmol (>1.2 mmol)
> Total cholesterol/HDL cholesterol ratio: 4.5 mmol (< 4.5 mmol)
> Triglycerides: 2.3 mmol (< 1.5 mmol)

As a student you should be able to interpret commonly used terms such as:

- hyperlipidaemia; raised levels of one or more of total cholesterol, LDL cholesterol or triglycerides
- combined hyperlipidaemia; hyperlipidaemia where both total cholesterol and triglycerides are raised
- dyslipidaemia; includes hyperlipidaemia and low levels of HDL cholesterol
- mixed dyslipidaemia; elevated levels of total cholesterol, LDL cholesterol

or triglycerides and low levels of HDL cholesterol. This is often associated with secondary causes such as diabetes or metabolic disease.

- familial dyslipidaemia; genetic conditions that predispose people to abnormal levels of lipids and include familial hypercholesterolaemia (grossly high levels of total cholesterol) and familial combined hyperlipidaemia (raised total cholesterol and triglycerides

**TABLE 7.2** OSCE marking criteria for explaining blood test results following a cholesterol test

| MARKING CRITERIA – BLOOD TEST RESULTS FOLLOWING A CHOLESTEROL TEST |
| --- |
| Student's general approach: introduces self, is warm and shows empathy |
| Student correctly explains blood test results in a language the patient understands |
| Student correctly identifies that the patient has hyperlipidaemia |
| Student checks the patient understands the result |
| Student explores lifestyle issues with the patient, e.g. smoking |
| Student discusses diet with the patient |
| Student discusses exercise with the patient |
| Student explains the importance of lifestyle changes in combination with cholesterol-lowering drugs |
| Student discusses treatment options with the patient, using evidence-based guidelines |
| Student correctly explains how the drug works |
| Student explains how to take the drug (including dosage and timing) |
| Student advises the patient of possible side effects |
| Student asks the patient to repeat what they have said to check the patient has understood |
| Student explores the patient's concerns |
| Student asks the patient if they have any questions |
| Student arranges for a follow-up appointment and repeat blood test |

Due to local drug policies and guidelines, it may be difficult to include exact reference ranges or treatment options in the marking criteria unless all the students undertaking the OSCE are from the same place. In reality, students have access to local drug policies, clinical guidelines, and the *British National Formulary*,[2] and so it would be reasonable to have them available for reference should they be required.

Our other conveying information example is for a patient who presents for the results of a liver function test. The scenario requires explaining the result to the patient and then exploring the underlying problem with the patient. This scenario does not require you to discuss the management and treatment options.

## OSCE scenario for altered liver function results

'A 43-year-old patient has presented to you today because she has recently had some blood tests taken by the locum nurse practitioner. The receptionist has asked the patient to come and see you to discuss the results.'

When you are ready, explain the result to the patient and explore the problem with her.

---

**Box 7.3  Scenario for a patient with liver function results**

You should not volunteer easily the fact that you have drunk alcohol daily for the last 13 years since your divorce. You drink on your own at least one bottle of wine a day and several vodkas. You sometimes begin to drink as early as 11 o'clock in the morning. You are not ready to accept that your recent feelings of being unwell are related to your drinking.

You have lost weight in the past 6 months but have had little appetite lately. You work as a freelance writer but find it increasingly difficult to work to deadlines – lack of money is now adding to your stress.

You do not have any children. Your father had an alcohol problem. You have no relevant medical history.

---

**Box 7.4  Patient's liver function blood test results**

| Haematology | Results | Measurement unit | Normal reference range |
|---|---|---|---|
| White blood cells | 9 | x 109/L | 5–18 |
| Red blood cells | 37 | x 1012/L | 5–98 |
| Haemoglobin | 10 | g/dl | 12–18 |
| Mean cell volume | 105 (high) | fl x10/L | 84–99 |
| Platelets | 321 | | 169–358 |
| **Biochemistry** | **Results** | **Measurement unit** | **Normal reference range** |
| Albumin | 83 | g/L | 30–52 |
| Alanine-amino transferase | 53 (high) | IU/L | 5–50 |
| Total bilirubin | 8 | IU mol/L | Up to 17 |
| Alkaline phosphatase | 180 | IU/L | 40–200 |
| Gamma-glutamyl transpeptidase | 348 (high) | U/L | (< 33) women<br>(< 51) men |

**TABLE 7.3** OSCE marking criteria for communicating blood test results following a liver function test

| MARKING CRITERIA – BLOOD TEST RESULTS FOLLOWING A LIVER FUNCTION TEST |
| --- |
| Student introduces self to patient |
| Student's general approach to the patient is warm and empathetic |
| Student explains the reason for blood test |
| Student explains the results clearly to the patient, using language that the patient understands |
| Student says that findings are abnormal |
| Student says that findings are likely to be the result of excessive alcohol |
| Student explores patient's use of alcohol showing sensitivity |
| Student explains the consequences of excessive use of alcohol |
| Student explains the pattern of alcohol use |
| Student discusses the implications of the blood results in terms of alcohol use |
| Student explains the safe level of alcohol use |
| Student explains the potential associated symptoms, e.g. loss of appetite, loss of weight, memory loss, etc. |
| Student discusses the patient's social circumstances, work and lifestyle issues |
| Student discusses the patient's past medical history, in relation to alcohol use |
| Student discusses the patient's work issues |
| Student discusses the patient's past medical history in relation to alcohol use |
| Student explores the patient's family history of alcohol abuse |
| Student explores the patient's readiness to change alcohol behaviour |
| Student discusses self-help support, e.g. Alcoholics Anonymous |
| Student discusses the availability of local services and support groups for alcohol and drug abuse |
| Student arranges support for the patient, e.g. referral for counselling |
| Student arranges a repeat liver function test in 3 months |

A further example of a conveying information OSCE station might be the interpretation of an investigation related to sexual health, such as a chlamydia positive test result.

## OSCE scenario for a patient presenting for the results of a swab test

'Sharon, a 21-year-old patient has come to see you today for the results of a chlamydia culture that was taken on her last visit with the practice nurse. The chlamydia result is positive.'

Please discuss the results with her, exploring relevant issues and management.

---

**Box 7.5 Scenario for a patient for chlamydia results**

Your name is Sharon and you are 21 years old. You have come to see the nurse practitioner today for the results of a chlamydia culture that you had on your last visit to the clinic. The nurse, who took it, suggested that this should be done, but you did not really understand why.

You are a single mother with one child, and have been in a new relationship for the last 3 months. Before that you were in a long-term relationship for 2 years. You have had no unusual symptoms that would indicate you have a sexually transmitted infection. You have used the contraceptive pill for 5 years and you have not had any problems. Your new boyfriend does not like using condoms.

You have heard of chlamydia before, from a magazine, but do not know much more about it. Your current partner has not complained of any signs or symptoms indicating sexually transmitted infection.

You would quite like to have more children at some point.

A friend of yours has had bacterial vaginosis and you think that this may be the same thing as chlamydia. You have never had a smear test. You are not allergic to anything that you know about. You are otherwise fit and well.

---

**TABLE 7.4** OSCE marking criteria for communicating the results of a chlamydia test

This station is primarily designed to test the student's competency and proficiency in communicating positive chlamydia laboratory results and discussing the implications with the patient.

| MARKING CRITERIA – RESULTS OF A CHLAMYDIA TEST |
| --- |
| Student introduces self, using a warm and empathetic approach |
| Student asks open-ended questions demonstrating sensitivity and good communication skills throughout |
| Student assesses patient's understanding of reason for swab being taken |
| Student assesses patient's current knowledge base about chlamydia and other sexually transmitted infections |
| Student explores patient's concerns and health beliefs |
| Student explains the result clearly, avoids medical jargon and pitches explanation at an appropriate level |
| Student checks the patient's understanding of chlamydia |

*(continued)*

---

MARKING CRITERIA – RESULTS OF A CHLAMYDIA TEST

---

Student asks whether the patient has a past history of sexually transmitted infections

Student explores signs and symptoms of chlamydia

Student asks about the patient's sexual relationships (stable, multiple partners)

Student asks about the patient's use of contraception, e.g. condoms

Student explains possible implications of chlamydia, e.g. pelvic inflammatory disease and infertility

Student asks about the date and result of the patient's last cervical smear

Student asks if the patient has any known allergies, e.g. to antibiotics

Student discusses management with patient, including antibiotics, e.g. doxycycline and emphasises compliance as per local protocol

Student discusses need for the patient's partner(s) to be tested/treated, and considers referring the patient to sexual health clinic

Student discusses contact tracing with the patient

Student discusses future prevention of transmission (e.g. protected intercourse)

Student advises patient to return for recheck test or if she experiences any problems with treatment

Student advises to return if any problems with prescribed treatment

---

## Treatment and management stations

These stations can be used to assess a student's ability to interpret a result and convey accurate information on the treatment and management of a prescribed situation. This could include both the pharmacological and the non-pharmacological knowledge required to manage the patient with the aim of establishing concordance.

## OSCE hypertension treatment and management

A 49-year-old Caucasian woman, Mrs Brown, was diagnosed with hypertension three months ago by her GP and given medication. She moved soon after and therefore cannot return to her original GP.

She has brought a note of the medication which says 'Ramipril 1.25 mg one tablet once a day'. She has come to see you for the first time today. Her blood pressure today is 162/110. Please explain to Mrs. Brown why she has been prescribed ramipril and the risk factors associated with high blood pressure.

The *British National Formulary*[3] and relevant evidence-based guidelines could be made available for you to use as a resource at this station.

## Box 7.6 Scenario for a patient with hypertension

You are Mrs. Brown, a 49-year-old Caucasian woman. You were diagnosed with hypertension three months ago by your GP. At the time he gave you a basic explanation of what hypertension was. He also gave you some medication which he said you must take and you took it for 1 month until the pills ran out. You have not taken any in the 2 months since. When you took them you did not notice any side effects.

You have come to see the nurse practitioner today as your neighbour said that you have to take blood pressure medication for life and you are now worried. You have brought a note of what your GP prescribed; this says Ramipril 1.25 mg one tablet once a day.

If asked you can mention that:

Your father had high blood pressure and died of a stroke (aged 72). Your brother also has high blood pressure (currently aged 52). You work in a supermarket near your new home. You quite enjoy it and do not find it stressful. You are married with two adult children who have left home. You have not exercised since teenage years.

You are *not* overweight. You stopped smoking 10 years ago – you used to smoke five to 10 cigarettes a day for 20 years. You drink two to three units of wine at the weekends only.

You think that you eat fairly healthily, although you like a lot of salt on your food.

You are not taking any other medication and do not have any outstanding medical conditions that you are aware of. Your blood test results were normal when you last had them taken at your GP, but you are not sure what they were for.

**TABLE 7.5** OSCE marking criteria for communicating hypertension treatment and management

| MARKING CRITERIA – HYPERTENSION TREATMENT AND MANAGEMENT |
| --- |
| Student introduces self to patient |
| Student uses verbal and non-verbal communication to encourage patient participation |
| Student uses reflection to ascertain the patient's understanding of the issues being discussed |
| Student uses language overall that the patient understands |
| Student elicits the patient's current health status/use of other medications |
| Student elicits the patient's past medical history |
| Student elicits the patient's family history of hypertension |

(*continued*)

---

**MARKING CRITERIA – HYPERTENSION TREATMENT AND MANAGEMENT**

Student asks about the patient's history of smoking

Student explains that the patient's BP reading today is higher than normal limits

Student explains what hypertension is

Student discusses the long-term consequences of untreated high blood pressure, especially increased risk of stroke

Student discusses the increased risk of cardiac disease, heart attack and angina

Student explains the increased risk of retinal haemorrhage

Student explains the increased risk of renal impairment

Student evaluates the patient's understanding of the advice

Student arranges a prescription for an appropriate anti-hypertensive treatment with reference to evidence-based guidelines

Student explains the potential side effects of the treatment

Student discusses other lifestyle factors to help reduce blood pressure along with medication
- diet (reduced intake of salt)
- exercise
- relaxation activities

Student discusses follow-up arrangements to monitor blood pressure and medication compliance

---

Laminated pictures can also be used in treatment and management OSCE stations to enable students to make an accurate diagnosis and then discuss the relevant treatment and management. The scenario for a skin condition is particularly suited to this type of OSCE station. This is useful to supplement the role-play, especially if no make-up is available. Some OSCEs may use real patients/actors with specific conditions, for example, eczema or psoriasis. This helps the OSCE to become more realistic but can be confusing for the students if they are not prepared for real patients. In this situation, care must be taken to ensure that the patient sticks to the written patient instructions and is not tempted to make up their own story.

## OSCE scenario for the treatment and management of a patient presenting with a skin infection

'Mrs Anderson is a 38-year-old woman who has come to see you today. You have not met her before.'

During this 10 minute station, you are required to take a history from the patient and discuss your diagnosis and management plan with the patient.

**TABLE 7.6** OSCE marking criteria for communicating the treatment and management of a skin infection

---

MARKING CRITERIA – TREATMENT AND MANAGEMENT OF A SKIN INFECTION

---

Student introduces self to patient

Student establishes rapport with patient

Student demonstrates structured history taking skills

Student asks open-ended questions

Student elicits
- provocative factors
- palliative factors
- quality of symptoms
- region of symptoms
- radiation of symptoms
- severity of symptoms
- timing of symptoms
- any other associated symptoms

Student elicits further information about
- allergies
- prescribed medication
- occupation
- over-the-counter medication
- remedies tried
- past medical history
- family history
- other family members with similar symptoms

Student asks about
- recent travel
- contraception
- hobbies
- pets
- smoking
- alcohol
- use of recreational drugs
- work concerns, e.g. time off

Student establishes differential diagnoses
- infected contact dermatitis/eczema
- trauma, e.g. burn
- infected insect bite (cellulitis)

Student discusses management
- wound dressing
- antihistamines
- antibiotic (for secondary infection)
- offers advice on hand care
- offers advice on work
- offers follow up appointment/referral

---

---

### OSCE stations that assess communication skills, conveying information, and treatment and management in summary

The key to success in these of type of OSCE stations is to try to ensure that you feel accomplished and comfortable (or at least can give an impression of being accomplished) in your professional interactions with patients and carers. The consultation communication skills that you use in your everyday clinical practice are equally applicable in these types of OSCE stations and they should be used accordingly. In support of your professional interactions you also need to have the background scientific knowledge related to the results of clinical investigations; this knowledge only comes from focused reading of the relevant medical literature accompanied by your interpretation of real clinical investigations in practice, supported by your supervising facilitator or mentor.

---

## References

1 Clinical knowledge summaries. *Depression.* Available at: http://cks.library.nhs.uk/depression (accessed 2 Jun 2008).
2 Martin J, Jordan B, Macfarlane C, *et al.*, editors. *British National Formulary 56.* London: BMJ Group and RPS Publishing; 2008
3 Martin, Jordan, Macfarlane, *et al.*, op. cit.

## Further reading

McGhee M. A *Guide to Laboratory Investigations.* 5th ed. Oxford: Radcliffe Publishing; 2008.
Neighbour R. *The Inner Consultation.* 2nd ed. Oxford: Radcliffe Publishing; 2005.

# 8

# Master's level assessment and the objective structured clinical assessment (OSCA)

## What is the objective structured clinical assessment (OSCA)?

In the preceding chapters we have dealt primarily with the OSCE as applied to undergraduate nurse practitioner preparation. However, nurse practitioner educational preparation is increasingly being offered on a postgraduate basis, most often as postgraduate diplomas or master's degrees, or occasionally as discrete stand-alone modules. A question arises as to how these courses should be differentiated from an undergraduate nurse practitioner course, not only by virtue of the higher academic attainment expected to be demonstrated by these students, but also in the nature of their assessment of advanced practice skills competence. This chapter presents a case study of the innovative modification of the OSCE process at London South Bank University to assess students' progress in the clinical component of the MSc Nurse Practitioner degree. While this modified OSCE process was developed at London South Bank University, we view this process as being readily transferable to other universities involved in assessing advanced practice competence at master's level.

In developing the masters level assessment at London South Bank University the advanced nurse practitioner teaching team sought to create an assessment that reflects the clinical complexity which students may encounter in their workplace, while concurrently assessing the distinctive masters level cognitive characteristics of critical analysis, synthesis and problem-solving. From a practical perspective in order to differentiate between the undergraduate OSCE and the postgraduate OSCE, the modified master's version has been called an objective structured clinical assessment (OSCA).

As previously discussed, the OSCE is an assessment of specific, well-defined clinical skills where students follow a pre-designated route of individual stations designed to assess discrete components of a consultation which require the use of advanced clinical practice skills. The OSCA builds on elements of the OSCE, but in contrast concentrates on a total patient consultation, which also assesses the students' underpinning clinical knowledge. By reflecting the components of a consultation, the OSCA requires students to demonstrate competence in a range of clinical skills essential for the advanced nursing role, such as communication and history taking, advanced physical examination skills, clinical decision-making, diagnostic reasoning, interpreting investigations and developing and negotiating a treatment and management plan. These components reflect the cognitive competencies, practice-related competencies and personal dynamism that have been typically attributed to a master's level performance in nursing.[1]

The OSCA is conceptualised as two long case stations consisting of five integrated components designed to reflect the potential diversity of patient assessment. Each case comprises a complex patient presentation which is marked against specific criteria considered essential for the advanced nursing role. This long case station is distinct from the multiple short stations that are typical of the conventional OSCE format we have presented in the preceding chapters.

The OSCA utilises a long case scenario to reflect a holistic patient assessment, which consists of five components per case, each discretely assessing the range of essential advanced clinical practice skills. Each student is allocated one hour in which to complete an OSCA case, and is required to complete two cases in order to pass the exam. These integrated stations have been designed to reflect the complexity of clinical presentations that advanced nursing students may encounter in their clinical areas. It is the effective management of this complexity, as well as the students' ability to articulate their understanding of the underlying pathophysiological processes, together with their ability to problem solve, that distinguishes this master's level clinical examination from other clinical examinations.

Below, we present an example of a long case scenario OSCA station, as developed at London South Bank University, for a patient presenting with shortness of breath.

There are five integrated OSCA components to be completed over 1 hour:

- Part 1 – history taking
- Part 2 – physical examination
- Part 3 – clinical reasoning
- Part 4 – investigations
- Part 5 – treatment and management.

## Part 1 History taking

### Box 8.1 Scenario for a patient with shortness of breath

You are an older Afro-Caribbean man who presents to the clinic complaining of shortness of breath and tiredness. Your opening statement is, 'I'm getting so breathless and I feel tired'. Your name is Bill Giles. Your address is 28 Tresco Road, London SE15 3JB. Your date of birth is 6 June 1944.

Please try to avoid volunteering information about yourself but do answer the student's questions fully. The student may ask more detailed questions about a particular symptom, e.g. shortness of breath, during the initial history taking or at a later stage in the consultation. If the student starts with an open-ended question such as 'how can I help you today?' or 'what do you think is the problem?' then please respond in general terms, such as:

○ 'I am worried about feeling short of breath'
○ 'I feel like I have no energy and I am breathless at times'
○ 'I'm not sure what is wrong but I usually have more energy and I'm not usually short of breath.'

Criteria to be included in scenario if asked:

#### Shortness of breath symptoms

You have been feeling short of breath for the last 3 months, but recently it has got worse and now you have to stop to catch your breath even on a short walk. Your breathing has become progressively worse over the last 3 months. Before you were able to walk to the pub (15 minutes away) without any problems, but now you are finding that any exertion is causing you to become breathless. You also find that you are not able to walk up to your flat without having to stop to catch your breath.

In the last week or so you have found that lying in bed makes the breathing worse so you have been sleeping in a chair at times. You have been waking up in the night very short of breath. You have never had to use inhalers. You have not experienced chest tightness or chest pain.

### Lack of energy symptoms

You feel as if you have no energy – you used to have lots. This has become a problem over the last 3 months. You tend to sleep quite a lot during the day at the moment as you are not sleeping well at night because of the breathing.

### Cough symptoms

You have a productive cough in the morning, but it gets better as the day goes on. You have coughed in the morning for years, but now it is worse. The sputum is white and frothy and there is lots of it – sometimes it is yellow. There is no blood in the sputum. You have tried some cough medicine that your wife bought for you – it has not made any difference.

### Current health

You have to get up in the night to pass urine (approx two to three times) and have some hesitancy, but you think that all men of your age have that problem. You have never had a problem with your bowels and nothing has changed. You have not been unwell recently – you cannot remember the last time you had a cold. You have not lost any weight recently, in fact you think that you are putting on weight as your tummy seems to be getting bigger. You have not lost any appetite.

You find that your ankles get very swollen after sitting in the chair. Sometimes your fingers also appear to be swollen. You do not have any night sweats

### Past medical history

High blood pressure diagnosed 10 years ago treated with atenolol 50 mg once daily for the last 5 years. You have regular blood pressure checks with the practice nurse. You take your blood pressure tablets every morning at the same time as your wife. You were immunised against TB as a child, you are up to date with other vaccinations. You have no known allergies.

### Family history

Your mother died of a stroke aged 67. She also had diabetes. Your father died of lung cancer aged 70.

### Personal and social history

You are a retired bus driver. You came to the UK as a child. You are married with five children, all of whom are grown up with their own families. You think that you have a good family network and have no real problems at the moment.

You smoke 10–20 cigarettes per day. You have smoked since you were 16 years old. This has not changed and you have not thought about giving up smoking. You live in a council-owned flat on the 3rd floor. There is no lift, and you have lived there for the last 30 years.

Your wife is alive and well. She also has high blood pressure and has recently been diagnosed with diabetes which is controlled on tablets. You like to walk or take the bus, you do not own a car. You walk to the pub three lunch times per week where you have a 'few' pints (two to three pints over a 2 hour period), lunch and play cards with friends you used to work with on the buses.

You do not do any other exercise. You like to watch the cricket on television and occasionally one of your sons will take you to the local cricket ground if the West Indies are playing. Your wife does all the cooking. You like to eat traditional Afro-Caribbean food, but occasionally eat out. There are no pets at home.

### Your concerns

You are worried that you may have cancer of the lung, like your father.

When the student has finished the history taking they are required to tell the examiner the multiple hypotheses/differential diagnoses generated at this stage and give a brief rationale for each.

**TABLE 8.1** OSCA part 1 marking criteria – history taking

| MARKING CRITERIA – HISTORY TAKING |
| --- |
| Student introduces self to patient |
| Student uses open-ended questions appropriately |
| Student allows the patient to explain signs and symptoms without interruption |
| **Presenting symptoms** |
| Student explores the dyspnoea symptom |
| Student explores the fatigue symptom |
| Student elicits why the patient has attended |
| Student elicits when the problem started |
| Student elicits if anyone else close to him has been ill with a similar problem |
| Student elicits provoking factors, e.g. exercise, recent upper respiratory tract infection, etc. |
| Student elicits relieving factors, e.g. rest |
| Student establishes the effect of the symptom on the patient's activities of daily living |
| Student asks if the patient has any other associated problems |
| Student asks if the patient has a cough |
| Student asks if there is sputum production |
| Student asks about the colour and amount of the sputum |

(*continued*)

## MARKING CRITERIA – HISTORY TAKING

### ▸❶▸ Red flags

Student asks if the sputum is bloodstained

Student asks about the patient's weight loss

Student asks about the patient's weight gain

Student asks about patient's ankle oedema

Student asks about any changes in the patient's appetite

Student asks about patient's night sweats

### Past medical history/family history

Student establishes the patient's past medical history

Student asks about the patient's family history

### Lifestyle/social history

Student asks about the patient's
- smoking
- alcohol
- exercise
- diet
- occupation/past occupation
- home circumstances

### Medication and allergies

Student asks about medications.

Student establishes concordance with any medications

Student asks about allergies

Student asks about any other associated symptoms, e.g. bowels, urine

Student elicits any self-help by the patient to date

Student establishes what the patient thinks is wrong

## Possible differential diagnosis and rationale at this stage

| POSSIBLE DIFFERENTIAL DIAGNOSIS | RATIONALE |
|---|---|
| Tuberculosis | |
| Bronchiectasis | |
| Acute bronchitis | |
| Asthma | |
| Chronic obstructive pulmonary disease | |
| Allergy | |
| Pneumonia | |
| Neoplasm | |
| Congestive heart failure | |
| Others that the student mentions | |

## Part 2 Physical examination

In this scenario the student is required to perform a physical examination of the respiratory and cardiovascular system and explain the procedure. If the student attempts to examine another system, please stop them, say that the findings in this system are normal and ask them to proceed with another system exam.

**TABLE 8.2** OSCA part 2 – physical examination marking criteria

| MARKING CRITERIA – PHYSICAL EXAMINATION |
| --- |
| Student introduces self to patient and explains procedure |
| Student asks for patient consent to proceed with the examination |
| Student asks patient to undress and ensures that patient is adequately exposed |
| Student washes hands or uses hand spray |
| Student says they will takes vital signs: blood pressure, temperature, pulse |
| Student observes the colour of the patient |
| Student checks the patient's fingers for signs of:<br>• smoking<br>• clubbing<br>• capillary refill<br>• hand temperature |
| **Physical examination of respiratory system** |
| Student inspects the patient's chest, observing and examining for:<br>• symmetry<br>• respiratory rate<br>• tracheal deviation<br>• shape of chest<br>• use of accessory muscles/retracted interspaces<br>• supraclavicular lymph nodes<br>• tenderness |
| Student checks chest expansion on either anterior or posterior chest |
| Student checks for tactile fremitus on anterior chest |
| Student checks for tactile fremitus on posterior chest |
| Student percusses anterior chest, comparing sides |
| Student percusses posterior chest, comparing sides |
| Student auscultates anterior chest, comparing sides |
| Student auscultates posterior chest, comparing sides |
| Student identifies any added breath sounds that might be heard, e.g. wheezes, crackles, rhonchi |
| **Physical examination of cardiovascular system** |
| Student inspects the patient's lower extremities for<br>• colour<br>• hair loss |

*(continued)*

**MARKING CRITERIA – PHYSICAL EXAMINATION**

Student inspects the patient's lower extremities for: (cont.)

- vascularities
- temperature
- oedema
- peripheral pulses

Student positions the patient correctly in supine position with bed head at 30°

Student assesses the patient's jugular venous pressure (states measurement in centimetres)

Student palpates the patient's carotid pulse

Student listens to the carotid pulse for bruits with bell of stethoscope

Student palpates the precordium for thrills

Student palpates the apical impulse

Student confirms the characteristics of apical impulse

If not felt in supine position, student asks the patient to roll onto his left side and feels again

Student auscultates the patient's heart at aortic, pulmonic, tricuspid and mitral areas with diaphragm of stethoscope

Student auscultates heart at aortic, pulmonic, tricuspid, and mitral areas with the bell of the stethoscope.

Special manoeuvre: student asks the patient to sit, lean forward, exhale completely, and stop breathing on expiration. Student listens along left sternal border and apex

Special manoeuvre: student asks patient to roll onto left side and listens at apex with bell of stethoscope

The examiner presents the physical examination findings to the student.

---

### Box 8.2 Physical examination findings for patient with shortness of breath

- Temperature 35.4C
- Blood pressure 135/92
- Pulse 92
- Respirations 25 per minute
- Body mass index 29
- Capillary refill – approx 6 seconds
- Hands and feet feel cold and look cyanosed
- Pitting ankle oedema
- Chest is barrel shaped
- Jugular venous pressure 4 cm
- Apex of heart felt at 6th intercostal space towards the mid-axilla line
- Sound 3 heart sound heard
- Widespread bilateral wheezes heard throughout the lung fields

---

## Part 3  Clinical reasoning and diagnosis

Student instructions for 2-part component.

1  Based on what you know about the patient, you are now required to tell the examiner which of your differential diagnosis you are going to accept and which you are going to refute, giving your rationale for these decisions.

2  You are now required to demonstrate your clinical reasoning skills. The examiner will ask you a series of general questions relating to the physical examination of the respiratory and cardiovascular systems which do not specifically relate to this patient's clinical findings.

### Accept or refute differential diagnoses with rationale

The student may need to be reminded of the differential diagnoses they generated after taking the history from the patient.

| DIFFERENTIAL DIAGNOSIS | RATIONALE | ACCEPTED | REFUTED |
|---|---|---|---|
| Tuberculosis | | | |
| Bronchiectasis | | | |
| Acute bronchitis | | | |
| Asthma | | | |
| Chronic obstructive pulmonary disease | | | |
| Allergy | | | |
| Pneumonia | | | |
| Neoplasm | | | |
| Congestive heart failure | | | |
| Others – please list those mentioned in part 1 | | | |

## Clinical reasoning questions

### 1 List three clinical signs evident on the patient's hands that suggest pathology in the respiratory or cardiovascular system

| CLINICAL SIGN (EXAMPLES OF ANSWERS) | MENTION |
| --- | --- |
| Clubbing | |
| Splinter haemorrhages | |
| Cyanosis | |
| Janeway's lesions | |
| Osler's nodes | |

### 2 Explain what the following findings on a respiratory exam may indicate

| CLINICAL FINDING | MENTION |
| --- | --- |
| Pleural rub: | |
| • pleurisy | |
| Crackles: | |
| • infection | |
| • pulmonary oedema | |
| Wheezes: | |
| • asthma | |
| • tuberculosis | |
| • tumour | |
| • infection | |
| • chronic obstructive pulmonary disease | |
| Rhonchi: | |
| • asthma | |
| • allergy | |
| • chronic obstructive pulmonary disease | |

### 3 List five physical examination findings that may indicate chronic obstructive pulmonary disease

| PHYSICAL EXAMINATION FINDING | MENTION |
| --- | --- |
| Rhonchi | |
| Tracheal tug | |
| Contraction of the sternomastoid muscle during inspiration | |
| Excavation of suprasternal and supraclavicular fossae during inspiration together with retraction of interspaces and costal margins | |
| Barrel chest | |

*(continued)*

| PHYSICAL EXAMINATION FINDING | MENTION |
|---|---|
| Weight loss | |
| Pursed lip breathing | |
| Central cyanosis | |
| Flapping tremor/bounding pulse | |
| Peripheral oedema | |
| Raised jugular venous pressure | |

## 4 Explain why a patient may have crackles in the lung fields if they have a diagnosis of pulmonary oedema

| EXPLANATION | MENTION |
|---|---|
| There is a rise in hydrostatic pressure due to an imbalance of fluid movement between the interstitial spaces (1*) | |
| As arterial pressure rises so does pulmonary venous and capillary pressure (1*) | |
| Pulmonary oedema occurs if the lymphatic system cannot cope with the fluid overload (1*) | |

* mark given for each explanation mentioned

## 5 List five clinical findings that may indicate right-sided heart failure

| CLINICAL FINDING | MENTION |
|---|---|
| Peripheral oedema | |
| Shortness of breath | |
| Hepatomegaly | |
| Splenomegaly | |
| Raised jugular venous pressure | |
| Ascites | |
| Slow weight gain | |
| Arrhythmias | |
| Abdominal distension | |
| Nausea | |
| Vomiting | |
| Anorexia | |
| Jaundice | |
| Weakness | |
| Fatigue | |
| Dizziness | |
| Syncope | |

## 6 Briefly explain the pathophysiology of the airways during asthma

| EXPLANATION | MENTION |
| --- | --- |
| Inhalation of an allergen causes an acute inflammatory response (*) with resulting broncho-constriction (*). | |
| Inflammatory mediators cause plasma exudation (*) to build up in the airways, resulting in mucous plugging, decreased mucociliary clearance, and oedema of the airway (*) causing airway obstruction (*). | |

* marked out of five. 1 mark given for each mentioned

## Part 4   Interpretation of investigations

1   The student is required to tell the examiner what are the most appropriate investigations that they would request for this patient.

2   The examiner will give the student some investigation results and the student is required to explain these results and their implications to the examiner.

3   Once the student has done this they are required to tell the examiner what they think the diagnosis is for this patient.

If the diagnosis is incorrect, the examiner will tell the student the correct diagnosis before they start part 5 of the OSCA

### Student's choice of investigations

| INVESTIGATION | MENTIONED |
| --- | --- |
| Full blood count | |
| Erythrocyte sedimentation rate | |
| Lipid profile | |
| Urea and electrolytes | |
| Liver function | |
| Glucose | |
| Thyroid function | |
| Chest X-ray | |
| Spirometry | |
| Peak flow | |
| Electrocardiogram | |
| Blood gases/oxygen saturation | |
| Others: | |

### Interpretation of three investigations relevant to the patient

The examiner gives the student three separate investigations to interpret, for example: an electrocardiogram, a chest X-ray and spirometry results.

| INVESTIGATION | CORRECT INTERPRETATION OF INVESTIGATION |
| --- | --- |
| Chest X-ray | |
| Spirometry | |
| Electrocardiogram | |

The diagnosis for this patient is chronic obstructive pulmonary disease with congestive cardiac failure.

## Part 5  Treatment and management

The student is now required to explain their diagnosis and treatment options to their patient, including appropriate pharmacological and non-pharmacological management and treatment.

The *British National Formulary* and clinical knowledge summaries guidelines are available to you for reference if needed.

**TABLE 8.3** OSCA part 5 – treatment and management marking criteria

| MARKING CRITERIA – TREATMENT AND MANAGEMENT |
| --- |
| Student explains purpose of discussion to patient |
| Student accurately explains diagnosis to patient: Chronic obstructive pulmonary disease is a disorder characterised by airflow obstruction, it is usually progressive, not usually reversible |
| Left sided heart failure is usually due to left ventricular dysfunction |
| Student explains the importance of giving up smoking |
| Student advises patient on how to give up smoking |
| Student explains the importance of losing some weight |
| Student discusses how the patient may lose weight |
| Student discusses chronic obstructive pulmonary disease management; initiates short-acting bronchodilator as needed (beta-2 agonist or anticholinergic) |
| Student explains how one of these drugs works |
| Student explains how to use this drug correctly |
| Student explains how to use a spacer |
| Student explains the side effects of the treatment<br>• beta 2-agonist<br>• fine tremor<br>• hypokalaemia<br>• anticholinergic: urinary retention in older men<br>• dry mouth |

*(continued)*

### MARKING CRITERIA – TREATMENT AND MANAGEMENT

Student explains that they will trial the above therapy for 4 weeks and then review it

Student explains heart failure management and discusses starting a relevant drug

Student explains reason to patient: the drug is the first line of treatment for a patients with heart failure and will also manage his blood pressure

Student explains how the selected relevant drug works

Student explains the need to titrate the drug

Student explains the side effects

- cough
- hypotension

Student explains the need to introduce a diuretic

Student explains how the drug works

Student explains when to take the drug

Student explores the need for follow-up visits

Student explains when to urgently refer to the clinic

Student gives the patient the opportunity to ask questions

---

### OSCA stations in summary

The above example is just one OSCA station. As can be seen, in this type of long case scenario, the station assesses and links a level of clinical complexity that is not always evident in more traditional short OSCE stations. OSCA-type stations require a large time commitment on the part of both students and academic staff for their respective planning, preparation, revision and performance. They may not therefore be relevant to every university or advanced nursing student, but they may be when a master's level of clinical complexity needs to be assessed.

## Reference

1 Ashworth P. Whither nursing? Discourses underlying the attribution of master's level performance in nursing. *J Adv Nurs.* 2001; 34(5): 621–8.

## Further reading

Ward H, Willis A. Assessing advanced clinical practice skills. *Primary Health Care.* 2006; 16(3): 22–4.

# 9

# Non-medical prescribing OSCEs

This chapter looks at another part of advanced practice; the developing field of non-medical prescribing, which is increasingly becoming an essential component of the advanced clinical practice of nurses, pharmacists and allied health professionals. We start by placing non-medical prescribing in its historical context, then provide examples of both university and practice-based nurse prescribing OSCEs, which students will find useful for their nurse independent prescribing OSCE preparation and revision.

## Contextual background of non-medical prescribing

Non-medical prescribing in the UK has been evolving at a slow and steady pace following the recommendation in 1986, by the Cumberlege Report, that nurses working in the community setting should be given prescriptive authority to prescribe from a limited formulary to provide a more efficient service to the patients they visit.[1] Following the 1992 Medicinal Products: Prescription by Nurses Act, limited prescribing rights were granted to health visitors, district nurses and practice nurses with a health-visiting or district nursing qualification.[2] Initially, programmes for educating nurse prescribers were integrated into the post-registration district nursing and health visitors' qualifications. Following much debate and lobbying from organisations such as the Royal College of Nursing, a consultation to extend nurse prescribing resulted in the 2001 Health and Social Care Act, which provided the necessary legislation to implement independent extended nurse prescribing. Nurses were then given the right to prescribe independently from an extended nurse-prescribing formulary.[3]

In May 2006 an important change in the prescribing regulations occurred when the extended formulary for nurse prescribers was discontinued and qualified nurse independent prescribers were permitted to independently prescribe any licensed medicine for any medical condition within their competence, including some controlled drugs. Alongside these advanced nursing developments pharmacists were granted supplementary prescribing rights in 2003 and independent prescribing rights in 2007. The allied health professions, including physiotherapists, podiatrists, radiographers and optometrists, were granted supplementary prescribing rights in 2006. These initiatives paved the way for the development of short stand-alone nurse prescribing programmes, offered as separate entities from other programmes for healthcare professional preparation. Most UK universities now offer programmes in non-medical prescribing, at either undergraduate or postgraduate certificate level.

In June 2006 the Nursing and Midwifery Council published its *Standards of Proficiency For Nurse and Midwife Prescribers*, which describes the statutory requirements for the education and training to prepare nurses to prescribe, the standards for prescribing practice, and additional practical guidance, such as writing a prescription.[4] The Nursing and Midwifery Council's education standard, which describes the requirements for assessing nurse independent and supplementary prescribers refers to the use of a practical assessment strategy demonstrating the application of prescribing theory to practice via an OSCE, either in a simulated learning environment (such as a university skills laboratory), or alternatively, in a practice setting relevant to a non-medical prescribing student's area of practice.[5] Beyond this requirement for either a university or practice-based prescribing OSCE assessment, there are no mandatory requirements for the number of OSCE stations or the nature of the stations to be undertaken on non-medical prescribing programmes. Accordingly there is a considerable variation in the number of OSCE stations used in non-medical prescribing programmes, with some universities using just one station, while others use up to 10.

## Non-medical prescribing OSCEs in a simulated learning environment

The Nursing and Midwifery Council has no currently laid down mandatory requirements regarding the format of non-medical prescribing OCSE stations, such as their timing and the exact prescribing competencies to be assessed in them. However each university needs to ensure that the advanced clinical skills of their non-medical prescribing students are assessed before they qualify as prescribers. The following examples are taken from the OSCE stations used on the non-medical prescribing programme at London South Bank University.

At London South Bank University the OSCE comprises of two stations. One is a 5 minute station and the other is a 10 minute station.

Several different types of 5 minute stations have been used at London South Bank University for the non-medical prescribing OSCEs. These have included staffed as well as unstaffed stations. The unstaffed stations do not have an examiner and a patient and the student is given a task can be completed in 5 minutes. The task to be completed at these unstaffed stations can vary to include activities such as writing a prescription, designing a clinical management plan or performing a drug calculation.

Like the OSCE stations described in previous chapters in this book, the staffed non-medical prescribing OSCE stations have both an examiner and a simulated patient. These stations commonly assess activities such as:

- safe prescribing and conveying information (5 minute station)
- taking a focused history of a common presenting complaint (5 minute station)
- history taking with linked diagnosis and management (10 minute station).

## Example of a safe prescribing and conveying information station

In this station the students are given a clinical scenario and a diagnosis. They are required to prescribe a correct dose of a given drug after having ascertained that it is safe for the patient to take that drug. The competencies assessed by this station include:

- communication skills
- ability to ask relevant questions to ensure the given drug is safely prescribed
- conveying appropriate information while prescribing the given drug.

Before the actual OSCE session, students are given a list of drugs that they could be tested on in the station. A *British National Formulary* is provided at the station for students to refer to if they need to.

The information given to the patient by the student should include:

- an explanation of patient's condition and how the prescribed drug will help them
- an enquiry about the cautions and contraindications for the drug (for example, pregnancy, breast-feeding, liver diseases, other drugs being taken etc.)
- information on any drug allergy
- an explanation of how to take the drug (dose, dose interval, duration)
- an explanation of the side effects of the drug.

## Example examination of a safe prescribing and conveying information OSCE station (from London South Bank University)

### Student instructions

Mrs Green, 32 years old is diagnosed as having acne.

She presents with inflammatory acne lesions on her back and you decide to prescribe tetracycline, 500 mg twice a day for two weeks. Explain to the patient what she needs to know about tetracycline. You can consult the *British National Formulary* provided at the station. You do not need to take a history. You will be assessed on your ability to do safe prescribing and convey drug information to the patient.

This is a 5 minute station.

**TABLE 9.1** OSCE marking criteria for safe prescribing and conveying information

| MARKING CRITERIA – SAFE PRESCRIBING AND CONVEYING INFORMATION |
| --- |
| Student gives appropriate introduction (their full name and clinical role) |
| Student explains that the patient has acne |
| Student explains that an oral antibiotic is needed for acne |
| Student enquires if Mrs Green is breast-feeding |
| Student enquires if Mrs Green is pregnant |
| Student explains the reason for asking about pregnancy and breast-feeding |
| Student asks about any other medications being taken; specifically over-the-counter, alternative medicines or any other drug being used |
| Student asks if the patient has any other medical ailments she knows of (liver disease, renal disease) |
| Student asks if the patient has any allergies |
| Student explains that tetracycline is an antibiotic being given for infection |
| Student explains that the patient will need to take 1 tablet twice a day for 14 days |
| Student advises the patient not to take the tablet with milk |
| Student cautions that there might be a stomach upset like, nausea, vomiting and diarrhoea due to the drug |
| Student explains that there can be reactions to the drug like rashes and reactions in the skin |
| Student advises the patient to report urgently if there is any headache or visual disturbance while taking the drug |
| Student advises regarding use of contraception while on medication |
| Student is well organised |
| Student uses clear, jargon-free language |
| Student checks the patient understands the advice |
| Student checks whether the patient has any questions |
| Student was empathetic and easy to talk with |

## Example of a focused history taking station (from London South Bank University)

In the 5 minutes provided, the student is required to take a focused history relating to the presenting complaint of the patient. The common complaints that the student could be assessed on include: pain (chest pain, musculoskeletal pain), fever, cough, itching (pruritus), headache, vomiting, diarrhoea or constipation.

### Student instructions

Mrs Janet Dela has come to your clinic. Please take a focused history of the presenting complaint. You do not need to take any history other than the history of present illness, which specifically is the detailed history of symptoms the patient presented with. You do not need to make a diagnosis or give management. This is a 5 minute station.

---

#### Box 9.1  Scenario for a patient with lower back pain

You are Janet Dela and you are 42 years old. You work as a freelance journalist. You are married. You have no children.

About a week ago you started having backache in your lower back. It was vague in nature. Initially you thought it would go but it has not improved. In fact, it has been worsening and you now have it all day. For the last two days you have not been able to do your daily morning exercise routine because of the pain.

The pain just seems to be there all day. It increases after you have been sitting in the same posture for more than half an hour. It also increases when you bend forward; so you have started to avoid bending forward due to the pain. It is not affected by ordinary breathing.

You have taken over-the-counter paracetamol tablets for the pain. Earlier, you needed to take two tablets and the pain would disappear for the whole day. Now, even with six tablets in a day, you feel the pain decreases but does not go away. For the past 3 days, you have not been able to sleep due to the pain. It is 7 on a scale of 1 to 10.

The pain does not radiate anywhere. There are no other symptoms. There has been no recent trauma to account for the pain. You do not drink alcohol. You smoke about 10 cigarettes a day and have been smoking since your teens. You have not noticed any change in your weight recently. You do not have any relevant past medical history, you do not regularly take any medicines, and you are not aware of having any allergies.

---

**TABLE 9.2** OSCE marking criteria for a focused history taking station with linked diagnosis for back pain

| MARKING CRITERIA – FOCUSED HISTORY TAKING STATION |
| --- |
| Student gives appropriate introduction (name and role) |
| Student asks about provoking factors (bending forwards, same posture) |
| Student asks about relieving factors (paracetamol) |
| Student asks about quality of pain (vague) |
| Student asks about radiation of pain (none) |
| Student asks about severity (asks on a numeric scale or asks with reference to interference with daily life due to pain) |
| Student asks about site of pain |
| Student asks about time of pain (duration and timing) |
| Student demonstrates good communication skills |
| Student demonstrates clear, structured history taking |
| Student uses open-ended questions. |
| This student made it easy for the patient to talk |

## General criteria for a history taking with linked diagnosis and management (from London South Bank University)

Here the student is required to choose the system that they would like to be tested on. This is designed to meet the learning needs of the student and reflect the area of practice in which they work. The range of systems that they can choose from include: dermatology, paediatrics, the gastrointestinal system, genital urinary medicine, the respiratory tract system, the cardiovascular system, or the musculoskeletal system.

The students are assessed on their:

- communication skills
- ability to take a detailed, structured history from the patient
- ability to make an appropriate diagnosis/differential diagnosis
- ability to provide suitable management advice to the patient.

The management advice could include:

- an explanation of the diagnosis to the patient
- any dietary/lifestyle advice or changes
- drugs that may be prescribed or a follow-up plan regarding drugs (this can include any plans for a clinical management plan or referral)
- safety netting
- a follow-up plan.

## Example of a history taking with linked diagnosis and management (from London South Bank University)

### Student instructions

Pat Field, 40, has come to see you in your minor illness clinic presenting with a 2-day history of diarrhoea and vomiting. This is the first time you have met.

You have 10 minutes to take a history, give a differential diagnosis and offer brief management advice. You will be told when you have 3 minutes before the end. It is advisable to start discussing the management at this point if you have not already done so.

**TABLE 9.3** OSCE marking criteria for a focused history taking station for diarrhoea

| MARKING CRITERIA – HISTORY TAKING WITH LINKED DIAGNOSIS AND MANAGEMENT |
| --- |
| Student introduces self (giving their name and role) |
| Student demonstrates good communication skills |
| Student demonstrates clear, structured history-taking |
| Student uses open questions |
| Student elicits when diarrhoea started |
| Student elicits when vomiting started |
| Student elicits frequency of stools now |
| Student elicits consistency of stools now |
| Student elicits whether there is any blood in the patient's stools |
| Student elicits whether there is any mucus in the patient's stools |
| Student elicits whether there is any pain in the patient's abdomen |
| Student elicits whether the patient is experiencing any abdominal bloating/flatulence |
| Student elicits whether there are any urinary symptoms |
| Student elicits whether the patient is experiencing any weight change |
| Student elicits any decrease in appetite or fluid intake |
| Student elicits past medical history |
| Student elicits whether any family members are involved |
| Student elicits whether the patient has undertaken any overseas travel |
| Student elicits the patient's occupation |
| Student elicits the patient's allergies |
| Student elicits the patient's last menstrual period |
| Student elicits the patient's contraception |
| Student elicits the patient's prescribed medication |
| Student elicits the patient's use of over-the-counter medication |
| Student elicits the patient's use of herbal medicines |

*(continued)*

| MARKING CRITERIA – HISTORY TAKING WITH LINKED DIAGNOSIS AND MANAGEMENT |
| :--- |
| Student suggests the patient has gastroenteritis |
| Student suggests the patient has a self limiting illness (average duration 5 days) |
| Student suggests the patient increases intake of fluids |
| Student suggests that the use of oral rehydration salts can be helpful, but this is mostly unnecessary in short, uncomplicated cases |
| Student suggests that taking a little food, as required, often helps settle nausea |
| Student suggests the patient buys loperamide over the counter |
| Student suggests the patient takes paracetamol 500 mg two tablets as required |
| Student suggests hand-washing for all family members |
| Student suggests safety netting if the patient is not improving or there is a worsening of their symptoms |
| This student makes it easy for the patient to talk |

## ►❿► Red flags in non-medical prescribing OSCE stations

Some non-medical prescribing OSCE stations may have pre-identified points on the marking sheet that are considered as essential to cover in the history. A failure to cover any of these red flags leads to the student failing the station. Some of these red flags may relate to patient safety. For example, failing to enquire about pregnancy if a student wishes to prescribe trimethoprim violates a red flag.

## Non-medical prescribing OSCEs in practice settings

Due to the diversity of students in a non-medical prescribing course (nurses of varied disciplines and specialities, pharmacists and allied health professionals), it is a challenge to ensure that the OSCE stations being taken by the students is within their area of competence. At London South Bank University the professional diversity of the students is managed by giving them physiological system-based choices for their history taking, and linked diagnosis and management OSCE. However, this diversity of choice has obvious logistical issues for the OSCE co-ordinator designing and conducting the examination and subsequent OSCE session.

As an alternative some universities feel that the best way to address this professional diversity is to assess students in their practice setting. Another advantage of this approach is that assessing students in settings they are familiar with may decrease their stress and anxiety. Accordingly, many universities now conduct their non-medical prescribing OSCEs in their students' practice settings.

Typically these practice-based non-medical prescribing OSCEs are conducted by the student's medical mentor, known as a designated medical practitioner. A real consultation with a consenting patient is used for the OSCE, most often towards the end of the student's practice experience. Dependent on the protocol of an individual university, a member of the academic team may or may not be present during the practice-based assessment.

## Student preparation for OSCEs in practice settings

To secure success in a practice-based OSCE you must ensure that:
- you are familiar with the requirements for assessment
- you select a patient with an appropriate presenting problem
- the patient gives informed consent for participating in the examination
- your designated medical practitioner also understands the requirements for assessment.

It is probably not a good idea to select a patient with a complex medical history or a potentially complex presenting complaint, as this may detrimentally affect your performance. For example, if you are working in primary healthcare, an example of an appropriate patient presentation to select, which is not overly complicated but still allows you to demonstrate prescribing competence, would be a younger woman presenting with symptoms suggestive of acute uncomplicated cystitis.

Before the commencement of the practice-based OSCE you should ensure that your designated medical practitioner has the relevant assessment documentation to hand, and that they are cognisant with the prescribing standards you have to meet to successfully complete the assessment.

---

### Non-medical prescribing OSCEs in summary

Non-medical prescribing OSCEs are a developing field of advanced clinical practice educational assessment. Due to the large number of universities providing non-medical prescribing programmes, and the diversity of students undertaking those programmes, it is difficult to provide guidance to students and staff that will always be applicable to their particular requirements. However, assessment and attainment in non-medical prescribing OSCEs should always reflect the national statutory standards for prescribing practice. These standards, such as those produced by the Nursing and Midwifery Council[6] and the Royal Pharmaceutical Society of Great Britain,[7] should always be referred to by both academics and students, when planning, preparing or revising for non-medical prescribing OSCEs.

---

## References

1 Department of Health and Social Security. *Neighbourhood Nursing: a focus for care.* London: HMSO; 1986.
2 Department of Health and Social Security. *Medicinal Products: Prescription by Nurses Act.* London: HMSO; 1992.
3 Department of Health. *Health and Social Care Act.* London: HMSO; 2001.
4 Nursing and Midwifery Council. *Standards of Proficiency for Nurse and Midwife Prescribers.* London: Nursing and Midwifery Council; 2006.
5 Nursing and Midwifery Council, op. cit.
6 Nursing and Midwifery Council, op. cit.
7 Royal Pharmaceutical Society of Great Britain. *Curriculum for the Education and Training of Pharmacist Supplementary Prescribers to become Independent Prescribers.* London: Royal Pharmaceutical Society of Great Britain; 2006.

## Further reading

Franklin P. OSCEs as a means of assessment for the practice of nurse prescribing. *Nurse Prescribing.* 2005; 3(1): 14–23.
McGavock H. *How Drugs Work.* 2nd ed. Oxford: Radcliffe Publishing; 2005.
McGavock H, Johnston D. *Treating Common Diseases.* Oxford: Radcliffe Publishing; 2007.

# Marking the OSCE

This concluding chapter considers the final part of the OSCE process: marking. Equitable and consistent marking of OSCE stations is essential to ensure parity of assessment for students. We believe it is helpful to draw a distinction between marking and scoring OSCEs. Scoring OSCE papers is a contemporaneous process undertaken by an OSCE examiner during an actual OSCE session, while OSCE marking is a post-OSCE session activity undertaken by the academic staff and their selected external examiner. In OSCE scoring the examiners fill in the marking criteria for an individual OSCE station, but they are not necessarily making a final judgment on the student's performance. In contrast, in OSCE marking the academic team examines from an overall perspective a student's OSCE performance, using the previously completed OSCE scoring to make a final judgement on that performance. This marking process can also be informed by comments from the examiner and patient received during a meeting held at the end of an OSCE session. Several different methods are available for scoring OSCEs and the subsequent marking. We first consider the scoring of OSCEs, followed by OSCE marking and the differences between using pass/refer marks and percentage marks. Finally, we discuss the use of more quantitatively orientated methods for OSCE scoring and marking.

## Scoring OSCE stations

The scoring tool used in the OSCE is a vital part of the related validity and reliability of the examination. A simple way of scoring the OSCE is to construct a checklist of criteria against which the examiner ticks 'done', 'not done' or 'omitted'. This type of OSCE scoring is sometimes referred to as a 'criterion rating' tool. However, it can be argued that criterion rating is too simple and does not allow the examiner to credit students who, in their opinion, perform well. In response to this criticism some universities have adopted a global rating OSCE score where the examiners judge whether a student's performance is either referred, borderline, a pass, a good pass or excellent. However, as the OSCE, as suggested in its name, is designed to be an objective assessment, the potentially subjective opinions of examiners when scoring and rating students' OSCE performances using a global rating system, may not increase the reliability or validity of the OSCE, as examiners may be influenced when a scoring a student's paper by extraneous factors, such as the student's appearance or demeanour. In our experience the influence of these extraneous variables on examiner scoring can be reduced by using a simple three-part criterion rating tool. At London South Bank University our criterion rating tool is as follows:

- done (correctly)
- not done correctly (attempted, but technique is not correct, or information given is not correct)
- omitted (not attempted or mentioned).

The examiners are advised that each criterion must be observed or heard to have been done correctly by the student, so as to be marked as 'done'. The role of the simulated patient in OSCE scoring is to support the examiner and to give feedback as to whether or not a procedure has been done correctly. For example, if the student causes the patient pain when examining their ear canal, this is marked as 'not done correctly'. However, when an examiner marks 'not done correctly' the reason for this score must be given in the examiner comments box. This requirement is put in place as the student must understand why they have been scored 'not done correctly', as they may be under the impression that the technique they used was correct, and may subsequently challenge the examiner's scoring.

It is the examiner's responsibility to correctly fill in the marking criteria and to:

- ensure that every criterion is assessed and the rating is noted with no gaps
- that mark sheets are completed and checked to ensure consistency across all students undertaking the station
- that their comments made are constructive, relevant and, importantly, impersonal as they should reflect a professionally neutral judgement.

## Marking OSCE stations

Once an OSCE session has been completed and all the individual exam papers have been scored by the examiners and carefully collated by the OSCE co-ordinator, the marking process can start. If an OSCE session has lasted all day then the marking will most often be undertaken the next day. Alternatively, if a session takes place in the morning, the marking can be undertaken in the succeeding afternoon. OSCE station marking is normally conducted by members of the academic team with the support of a previously selected OSCE external examiner, who should have critically observed the OSCE session from which the exam papers to be marked arise. The external examiner is invited to participate in a review of each student's performance and to ensure that the decision-making process is objective, transparent and consistent. Each station is considered separately, and the assembled panel makes a collective final decision on whether a student passes or is referred in each station. The overall OSCE session profile for each student is then collated and the recommended outcome noted for subsequent consideration at the next university exam board.

Depending on the number of OSCE stations to be marked, team members can be allocated a set number of stations to review and check the scoring. The purpose of this review is to establish whether a student has achieved the requisite competency and safety standard to pass the station. One quick and effective way of identifying a student's demonstrated competency and safety for passing an OSCE session is to categorise some of the marking criteria as essential criteria, for which a positive score must be elicited in order to pass the station. These essential criteria can be linked to red flags. If a particular OSCE station scenario contains red flag criteria then the essential marking criteria should reflect this. Red flags are used to maintain patient safety. Thus when you establish essential marking criteria you may be laying out the rules for a student to be referred at a station for not asking the red flag questions, despite their meeting the station's other criteria. From a practical perspective in the marking process, the essential criteria and related scores on students' papers can be easily identified by the academic team by highlighting the relevant criteria with a highlighter pen. We have found it beneficial to allow only the academic team members to know the essential marking criteria for individual stations, as prior knowledge of these criteria may bias examiners' scoring of stations. They may, understandably, just focus on the essential criteria at the expense of the other criteria and of providing an evaluation of the students' overall performance.

Below we show an example of marking criteria for an adult female abdominal pain with dysuria history taking station, with the essential marking criteria highlighted*. In this case example the student would need to successfully score 'done' in all the essential marking criteria identified in order to pass the station. This is the minimum requirement for passing the station.

**TABLE 10.1** History taking OSCE station with essential criteria highlighted*

| MARKING CRITERIA SHOWING ESSENTIAL CRITERIA | DONE CORRECTLY | NOT DONE CORRECTLY | OMITTED |
|---|---|---|---|
| Student's general approach to patient: introduction, warmth, and empathy | | | |
| Student asks open-ended questions demonstrating sensitivity and appropriate communication skills throughout | | | |
| *Student determines patient's presenting complaint (abdominal pain and dysuria) | | | |

**Symptom analysis using OPQRST framework**

*Student asks about other symptoms
- frequency
- urgency
- nocturia
- unusual vaginal discharge
- vaginal/vulval irritation, spots or sores

*Student asks about provoking factors: *abdominal pain increases with micturition

Student asks about quality/quantity of abdominal pain: intermittent pain

Student asks about relieving factors
- abdominal pain
- partial relief with paracetamol

Student asks about region/radiation: suprapubic abdominal pain, no back pain

*Student asks about recurrence and whether the patient has had similar problems in the past.

Student asks about the severity of the problem: uses a pain-rating scale to assess severity of abdominal pain/dysuria, effect on life, e.g. time off work

*Student asks about timing: how long ago did the abdominal pain start, duration of dysuria, duration of other urinary symptoms

➤⬤➤ *Student asks about red flags symptoms
- *nausea and vomiting
- *haematuria
- *fever
- *possibility of pregnancy and last menstrual period
- history of abdominal or back trauma
- weight loss

*(continued)*

| MARKING CRITERIA SHOWING ESSENTIAL CRITERIA | DONE CORRECTLY | NOT DONE CORRECTLY | OMITTED |
|---|---|---|---|
| Student asks about the patient's | | | |
| • lifestyle | | | |
| • exercise | | | |
| • occupation | | | |
| • travel history | | | |
| Student asks about the patient's | | | |
| • *past medical history | | | |
| • any history of previous abdominal problems, such as cystitis | | | |
| • *drug history | | | |
| Student asks if any over-the-counter medicines have been tried and their effect | | | |
| *Student asks about allergies | | | |
| Student asks if the patient smokes or has ever smoked | | | |
| Student asks about the patient's weekly alcohol intake | | | |
| Student asks about the patient's sexual health history: Does she currently have a partner? Does she any new sexual contacts? When was her last sexual health screen? | | | |
| Student explores the patient's perceptions of what the problem is | | | |
| Student asks the patient what they would like to do about the problem | | | |
| Student demonstrates a structured approach to focused history taking | | | |

## Pass marks for OSCEs

The pass mark for the OSCE constitutes an academic debate as well as a challenge, as it can be argued that the standard 40% pass mark at undergraduate level and 50% at masters level is not applicable in an OSCE, as what is being assessed is clinical competence, not academic attainment. Some universities prefer a pass/refer mark for their OSCEs. London South Bank University has a preference for using the pass/refer mark, as we believe that this most realistically reflects clinical competence. However, other universities prefer to convert OSCE scores in percentage marks, like those awarded for written examinations or essays. The difference with an OSCE percentage mark over a written assessment percentage mark is that normally the threshold for scoring an OSCE pass is often increased to a higher level, such as 70%. However, we wonder whether a student can be 70% competent in their clinical perform-ance. As we do not think that this is a coherent position, we prefer using a simple pass/refer marking scheme, with related pre-identified essential criteria, which we think provides a more accurate assessment of demonstrated clinical competence in an OSCE.

Some advanced nursing academics believe that students' demonstrated clinical competence should be rewarded in percentage marks, which can then contribute to their overall degree classification in conjunction with their normal academic unit attainment. However as OSCE percentage mark scores are often placed at a relatively high level, such as the previously mentioned 70%, the inclusion of such high marks could artificially skew a student's degree classification upwards, while potentially masking poor marks in their written components of assessment.

The application of OSCE pass/refer criteria does not have to be used in isolation; it too can be related to academic attainment. This relationship can be developed by linking an identified OSCE session that a student needs to complete to one of the academic units in their advanced nursing programme of study. This means that if a student is unsuccessful in their OSCEs the mark for the related unit can be capped at the minimum pass mark of 40% (undergraduate) or 50% (postgraduate). This linkage of the OSCE to the academic unit means that underperformance in the OSCEs is reflected in academic marks attainment, while success in the OSCEs still contributes to the award of academic credit, but not through artificial grade inflation.

## Converting an OSCE score to a percentage mark

As an example, in a station with 23 different criteria a student might score 18/23 done correctly criteria. The following percentage calculation formula is used:

18 divided by 23 equals 0.782608

0.782608 multiplied by 100 equals 78.260 (which can be rounded up or down accordingly)

The percentage score for this station will then be 78%.

The overall percentage pass mark must be decided upon before the OSCE. A student's overall percentage for the total exam can be calculated, thus enabling the high scores at some of the OSCE stations to compensate for the low scores at others. For example, if the OSCE consists of five different OSCE stations, five percentages would be calculated, and it would be the mean percentage that is the overall mark for the student. If the pass mark is 70% then it would be possible for the student to score less than 70% in some stations and more than 70% in others, and if their overall mean percentage is over 70%, then the student could still pass the OSCE. However, the usage of this type of percentage marking does mean that the attainment of red flag essential criteria does not always need to be achieved by the student, as the overall percentage marking system may mask poorer aspects of the student's performance.

To remedy this situation some universities use OSCE percentage marking which incorporates a negative marking scheme, whereby essential red flag criteria are marked negatively (by a pre-determined deduction of marks) if done incorrectly or omitted, leading to the overall subtraction of percentage marks, which would then more realistically reflect a student's performance.

## The number of OSCE stations to be passed in an OSCE session

At London South Bank University in the final-year 10 station OSCE session the students must pass nine out of ten stations to pass the OSCE. If they pass eight out of ten stations, they are referred in the OSCE, and are required to retake a similar type of station (but not exactly the same one) at a date to be determined by the university examination board. If the students fail three or more stations they have to undertake the whole OSCE session again at the next occurrence of the OSCEs in the following academic year.

First-year introductory OSCEs can either be presented as formative assessments where the focus is on constructively developing the students' OSCE skills, rather than just on passing the examination. Alternatively, introductory OSCEs can be presented as summative assessments, allaying student anxieties by an OSCE referral process so that that the student is offered another OSCE attempt, but would have to repeat only the previous content of their referred station or stations. In effect, this would mean that the introductory OSCE retake would become a seen exam, which should make it relatively easy to pass, and hence help the students feel more comfortable about their impending OSCEs.

## Using video recording of OSCE stations for scoring and marking

Some universities have adopted a video-marking scheme which enables the academic team themselves to directly score and mark the OSCE stations objectively against the predetermined marking criteria. In this method the student's OSCE station performances are video recorded and are scored and marked once the recording of the whole OSCE session has been completed. The advantage of this method is that if the marker is not sure whether they have heard or seen a procedure then the recording can be watched again. The disadvantages are that the camera may not be able to pick up all the skills being examined, as a student may have their back turned to the camera, and the simulated patient may not always be able to feed back any discomfort to the marker, as the OSCE scoring will not be simultaneous, but instead occurs after the event.

## Using quantitatively orientated methods for OSCE scoring and marking

More explicit quantitatively orientated methods can be used for OSCE marking. These are particularly useful for making a judgment on borderline pass or referred OSCE candidates. In this borderline method the pass mark for an OSCE station is determined after the examination by calculating the average marks scored at a station by all the students classified as borderline by the examiner. This average mark is then used as the pass mark for that OSCE station.[1]

Some universities have adopted a modified borderline method for OSCE standard setting. This is similar to the borderline method, except that, following the calculation of a mean borderline score for each OSCE station, the total examination pass score is calculated by summing the pass marks for each station and finding the mean.

At London South Bank University for our non-medical prescribing OSCEs we use the borderline method for OSCE standard setting. At the bottom of each OSCE mark sheet there is an overall rating score that the examiner needs to give to the student based on their objective assessment. The examiners mark the students as either a clear pass (acceptable), a clear refer (unacceptable) or borderline. In order to minimise the inter-examiner variability in marking the overall scores, there are pre-indicated points on the OSCE mark sheet that are defined as critical points (similar to the red flag essential criteria). These are generally the points on the mark sheet that should be covered by the students to ensure safe prescribing, for example, asking about allergies before prescribing. The examiners are asked to mark a student as borderline or 'C' (cause for concern) if the student fails to cover any of the critical points, or if the student is neither a clear pass nor a clear fail, in the objective judgement of the examiner.

Following the OSCE session all the mark sheets of the borderline students are collated for each station. The passing score of the whole group for an OSCE station is then calculated by taking the average score for all the students with borderline performance on that station.

As an example, consider the mark sheet in Table 10.2. The total possible maximum score on the mark sheet is 13. At the bottom of the mark sheet is a space for the examiner to indicate their global rating for the candidate as A (acceptable/pass), C (cause for concern/borderline) or U (unacceptable/fail). Let us assume that 100 students appeared for the station and the examiner assessed 10 students as borderline. The marks obtained by the borderline students are presented in Table 10.3. The calculated mean of the marks by the borderline students is 10. Thus the passing mark for this station will be 10/13 on the mark sheet score.

**TABLE 10.2** OSCE quantitative style scoring scheme

| | | | |
|---|---|---|---|
| Student gives appropriate introduction (name and role) (1 point for each) | 2 | 1 | 0 |
| *Student enquires about the main symptom enquiry* | | | |
| Student enquires about provoking factors (bending forwards, same posture) | 1 | | 0 |
| Quality of pain (vague) | 1 | | 0 |
| Student enquires about relieving factors (paracetamol) | 1 | | 0 |
| Student enquires about radiation of pain (none) | 1 | | 0 |
| Student enquires about severity (asks on a numerical scale or asks with reference to interference with daily life due to pain) | 1 | | 0 |
| Student enquires about site of pain | 1 | | 0 |
| Student enquires about time of pain (duration and timing) | 1 | | 0 |
| *General* | | | |
| Good communication skills demonstrated | 1 | | 0 |
| Clear, structured history taking | 1 | | 0 |
| Open questions used | 1 | | 0 |
| (For the patient to comment on) This student made it easy for me to talk | 1 | | 0 |
| Overall rating (Acceptable, Cause for concern, Unacceptable) | A | C | U |

**TABLE 10.3** Marks obtained by the students graded as 'borderline'

| MARK SHEET SCORE | |
|---|---|
| Student 1 | 10 |
| Student 2 | 11 |
| Student 3 | 11 |
| Student 4 | 9 |

(*continued*)

| MARK SHEET | SCORE |
|---|---|
| Student 5 | 12 |
| Student 6 | 10 |
| Student 7 | 10 |
| Student 8 | 10 |
| Student 9 | 9 |
| Student 10 | 8 |
| Total score | 100 |
| Mean score (Total score/10) | **10** |

### Enumerated OSCE criterion rating categories

If so desired for alternative OSCE marking schemes, it is also possible to convert the previously mentioned OSCE scoring categories of 'done correctly', 'not done correctly', and 'omitted' into a similarly quantitatively orientated style. To create this further level of detail the categories should be enumerated, which gives a quantitative dimension to a student's OSCE performance as shown below:

- done correctly (score 2)
- not done correctly (score 1)
- not done at all/omitted (score 0).

In the example above done correctly equates with 'acceptable', not done correctly with 'cause for concern', and 'omitted' with 'unacceptable'. Once enumerated, the OSCE scoring categories can be quantified as in the borderline method discussed above for OSCE standard setting.

---

**OSCE marking in summary**

There is no gold standard method for scoring and marking OSCEs. Each method has its advantages and disadvantages. However, it is vital that the marking process used is evidence-based, feasible and transparent, and produces defensible outcomes. The ultimate aim of any method used for OSCE scoring and marking is to ensure a consistent and equitable assessment of students' OSCE performances, which uniformly rewards them for demonstrating advanced clinical practice competence.

---

### Reference

1 Wilkinson T, Newble D, Frampton C. Standard setting in an objective structured clinical examination: use of global ratings of borderline performance to determine the passing score. *Med Educ.* 2001; 35(11): 1043–9.

# Index